全国高等中医药院校中药学类专业双语规划教材
Bilingual Planned Textbooks for Chinese Materia Medica Majors in TCM Colleges and Universities

药剂学实验

Pharmaceutics Experiment

（供中药学类、药学类、制药工程及相关专业使用）
(For Chinese Materia Medica, Pharmacy, Pharmaceutical Engineering and other related majors)

主　编　韩　丽

副主编　王文苹　郑　琴　彭海生　谢兴亮　颜　红

编　者（以姓氏笔画为序）

王文苹（云南中医药大学）　　伍振峰（江西中医药大学）

孙　黎（安徽中医药大学）　　李　文（成都中医药大学）

李英鹏（天津中医药大学）　　邹俊波（陕西中医药大学）

张金秋（大庆师范学院）　　　张定堃（成都中医药大学）

陈桐楷（广州中医药大学）　　陈新梅（山东中医药大学）

郑　琴（江西中医药大学）　　彭海生（哈尔滨医科大学）

韩　丽（成都中医药大学）　　储晓琴（安徽中医药大学）

谢兴亮（成都医学院）　　　　蔡邦荣（河南中医药大学）

颜　红（湖南中医药大学）

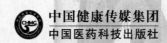

中国健康传媒集团
中国医药科技出版社

内容提要

本教材是"全国高等中医药院校中药学类专业双语规划教材"之一，包括两个模块共27个实验。在"制剂基础性实验"模块，按照药剂学教学大纲的要求及2020年版《中国药典》制剂通则的规定，从剂型、制备技术、质量三个方面，精选了有关普通剂型、新剂型、制剂新技术、稳定性等共19个实验，使学生通过实验操作系统验证、巩固和掌握药剂学基本理论知识；针对药剂学具有工艺学的性质，本书专列了"制剂评价技术"模块，设计了制剂工艺环节的7个相关参数检测实验，使学生更好地理解药剂的成型原理与质控方法，这部分内容是对药剂学实验的延伸和创新；另外，为适应创新性人才培养需求，在"制剂基础性实验"模块中安排了1个设计性试验，以培养学生分析问题、解决问题的能力及创新能力，为将来从事药物制剂的生产、新产品的研发奠定基础。

本教材供全国高等医药院校中药学类、药学类、制药工程及相关专业使用，也可供从事药物研究、生产、销售工作的人员参考。

图书在版编目（CIP）数据

药剂学实验：汉英对照 / 韩丽主编 . —北京：中国医药科技出版社，2020.9

全国高等中医药院校中药学类专业双语规划教材

ISBN 978-7-5214-1876-7

Ⅰ.①药… Ⅱ.①韩… Ⅲ.①药剂学 – 实验 – 双语教学 – 中医学院 – 教材 – 汉、英 Ⅳ.① R94-33

中国版本图书馆 CIP 数据核字（2020）第 097267 号

美术编辑 陈君杞

版式设计 辰轩文化

出版 **中国健康传媒集团** | 中国医药科技出版社

地址 北京市海淀区文慧园北路甲 22 号

邮编 100082

电话 发行：010-62227427 邮购：010-62236938

网址 www.cmstp.com

规格 889×1194 mm $\frac{1}{16}$

印张 13$\frac{1}{2}$

字数 356 千字

版次 2020 年 9 月第 1 版

印次 2020 年 9 月第 1 次印刷

印刷 三河市万龙印装有限公司

经销 全国各地新华书店

书号 ISBN 978-7-5214-1876-7

定价 48.00 元

获取新书信息、投稿、为图书纠错，请扫码联系我们。

近些年随着世界范围的中医药热潮的涌动，来中国学习中医药学的留学生逐年增多，走出国门的中医药学人才也在增加。为了适应中医药国际交流与合作的需要，加快中医药国际化进程，提高来中国留学生和国际班学生的教学质量，满足双语教学的需要和中医药对外交流需求，培养优秀的国际化中医药人才，进一步推动中医药国际化进程，根据教育部、国家中医药管理局、国家药品监督管理局等部门的有关精神，在本套教材建设指导委员会主任委员成都中医药大学彭成教授等专家的指导和顶层设计下，中国医药科技出版社组织全国 50 余所高等中医药院校及附属医疗机构约 420 名专家、教师精心编撰了全国高等中医药院校中药学类专业双语规划教材，该套教材即将付梓出版。

本套教材共计 23 门，主要供全国高等中医药院校中药学类专业教学使用。本套教材定位清晰、特色鲜明，主要体现在以下方面。

一、立足双语教学实际，培养复合应用型人才

本套教材以高校双语教学课程建设要求为依据，以满足国内医药院校开展留学生教学和双语教学的需求为目标，突出中医药文化特色鲜明、中医药专业术语规范的特点，注重培养中医药技能、反映中医药传承和现代研究成果，旨在优化教育质量，培养优秀的国际化中医药人才，推进中医药对外交流。

本套教材建设围绕目前中医药院校本科教育教学改革方向对教材体系进行科学规划、合理设计，坚持以培养创新型和复合型人才为宗旨，以社会需求为导向，以培养适应中药开发、利用、管理、服务等各个领域需求的高素质应用型人才为目标的教材建设思路与原则。

二、遵循教材编写规律，整体优化，紧跟学科发展步伐

本套教材的编写遵循"三基、五性、三特定"的教材编写规律；以"必需、够用"为度；坚持与时俱进，注意吸收新技术和新方法，适当拓展知识面，为学生后续发展奠定必要的基础。实验教材密切结合主干教材内容，体现理实一体，注重培养学生实践技能训练的同时，按照教育部相关精神，增加设计性实验部分，以现实问题作为驱动力来培养学生自主获取和应用新知识的能力，从而培养学生独立思考能力、实验设计能力、实践操作能力和可持续发展能力，满足培养应用型和复合型人才的要求。强调全套教材内容的整体优化，并注重不同教材内容的联系与衔接，避免遗漏和不必要的交叉重复。

三、对接职业资格考试，"教考""理实"密切融合

本套教材的内容和结构设计紧密对接国家执业中药师职业资格考试大纲要求，实现教学与考试、理论与实践的密切融合，并且在教材编写过程中，吸收具有丰富实践经验的企业人员参与教材的编写，确保教材的内容密切结合应用，更加体现高等教育的实践性和开放性，为学生参加考试和实践工作打下坚实基础。

四、创新教材呈现形式，书网融合，使教与学更便捷更轻松

全套教材为书网融合教材，即纸质教材与数字教材、配套教学资源、题库系统、数字化教学服务有机融合。通过"一书一码"的强关联，为读者提供全免费增值服务。按教材封底的提示激活教材后，读者可通过PC、手机阅读电子教材和配套课程资源（PPT、微课、视频等），并可在线进行同步练习，实时收到答案反馈和解析。同时，读者也可以直接扫描书中二维码，阅读与教材内容关联的课程资源，从而丰富学习体验，使学习更便捷。教师可通过PC在线创建课程，与学生互动，开展在线课程内容定制、布置和批改作业、在线组织考试、讨论与答疑等教学活动，学生通过PC、手机均可实现在线作业、在线考试，提升学习效率，使教与学更轻松。此外，平台尚有数据分析、教学诊断等功能，可为教学研究与管理提供技术和数据支撑。需要特殊说明的是，有些专业基础课程，例如《药理学》等9种教材，起源于西方医学，因篇幅所限，在本次双语教材建设中纸质教材以英语为主，仅将专业词汇对照了中文翻译，同时在中国医药科技出版社数字平台"医药大学堂"上配套了中文电子教材供学生学习参考。

编写出版本套高质量教材，得到了全国知名专家的精心指导和各有关院校领导与编者的大力支持，在此一并表示衷心感谢。希望广大师生在教学中积极使用本套教材和提出宝贵意见，以便修订完善，共同打造精品教材，为促进我国高等中医药院校中药学类专业教育教学改革和人才培养做出积极贡献。

全国高等中医药院校中药学类专业双语规划教材
建设指导委员会

数字化教材编委会

主　编　韩　丽

副主编　王文苹　郑　琴　彭海生　谢兴亮　颜　红

编　者　（以姓氏笔画为序）

王文苹（云南中医药大学）　　伍振峰（江西中医药大学）

孙　黎（安徽中医药大学）　　李　文（成都中医药大学）

李英鹏（天津中医药大学）　　邹俊波（陕西中医药大学）

张金秋（大庆师范学院）　　　张定堃（成都中医药大学）

陈桐楷（广州中医药大学）　　陈新梅（山东中医药大学）

郑　琴（江西中医药大学）　　彭海生（哈尔滨医科大学）

韩　丽（成都中医药大学）　　储晓琴（安徽中医药大学）

谢兴亮（成都医学院）　　　　蔡邦荣（河南中医药大学）

颜　红（湖南中医药大学）

药剂学是研究药物制剂的基本理论、处方设计、制备工艺、质量控制及合理应用的一门应用技术学科。药剂学实验的目的在于验证、巩固药剂学基本理论和知识，培养学生的专业技能和实践素质，为将来从事药物制剂的生产、研发奠定基础。

药剂学实验教材按照教学大纲，结合2020年版《中华人民共和国药典》（以下简称《中国药典》）标准要求，采用"制剂基础性实验"与"制剂评价技术"两个相互关联的模块，有区别、有层次地安排了27个实验项目，突出了药剂学学科的工艺学性质，体现了课程的系统性与实用性。

"制剂基础性实验"模块包括普通制剂、制剂新技术与新剂型、制剂稳定性、设计性试验等内容，共20个实验，内容涵盖液体、固体、半固体等剂型，体现了药剂学以剂型为中心的学科性质；制剂新技术、新剂型及综合设计性实验，旨在培养学生的分析问题能力和设计能力，适应创新性人才的培养需求。"制剂评价技术"模块安排7个实验，侧重于制剂成型过程中不同物态相关参数的测定及评价，使学生更好地理解药剂的成型机制及控制方法。

每一个实验的项下包括6个部分：实验目的、实验原理、实验器材、实验方法、实验结果与讨论、思考题。实验内容经过精心筛选，可操作性强。

本教材的英文翻译及专业术语的表达，主要参考了《中国药典》2015年版英文版，同时也参考了英文版药剂学教材及相关专业论文要求。双语形式有助于学生积累英语专业词汇和提升英语阅读能力，为以后论文撰写奠定基础，另一方面也有利于提升参与对外交流与合作的能力。

本教材是由从事药剂学教学与科研工作的骨干教师共同编写，全书英文修编由张金秋老师完成。在编写过程中，得到了各编者所在院校的大力支持，在此一并表示感谢。

本教材适用于中药学、药学、制药工程及相关专业的本科实验教学。

由于受编者水平所限，在内容安排和英文表述方面的不足之处在所难免，敬请广大读者提出宝贵意见和建议。

编者
2020年4月

Preface

Pharmaceutics is an applied and technical subject which studies the basic theory, formulation design, preparation process, quality control and reasonable application of pharmaceutical preparations. The purpose of pharmaceutical experiments is to verify and strengthen the theories and knowledge of Pharmaceutics, to cultivate the professional skills and practical ability of students, to lay the foundation for engagement in the production, research and development of pharmaceutical preparations in the future.

In accordance with the syllabus and the *Pharmacopoeia of the People's Republic of China* (2020), the textbook of *Pharmaceutics Experiment* is presented as two interrelated modules of "Basic experiments of pharmaceutical preparations" and "Evaluation technologies of pharmaceutical preparations", which contain 27 experiments to highlight the technological nature of pharmaceutics, and to reflect the systematization and practicability of the course.

The first module provides 20 experiments for common preparations, novel technologies and new dosage forms, preparation stability and design. The content involves a variety of liquid, solid or semi-solid dosage forms, which reflects the disciplinary characteristics of pharmaceutics centered on dosage form. The experiments on novel technology, new dosage forms and experiment design are aimed to cultivate students' analyzing and problem-solving capability, and to meet the demands of innovative talents. Seven experiments are listed in the second module, which mainly focus on the measurement and evaluation of related parameters for different physical states during the formulation process, so that students can better understand the formation mechanism of pharmaceuticals.

Each experiment includes six parts: objectives, principles, equipments and materials, methods, results and discussions as well as questions. These experiments are carefully selected and easy to operate.

The English translation and the expression of professional terminology mainly refer to the English edition of *Pharmacopoeia of the People's Republic of China* (2015), the English version of pharmacy textbooks and related professional paper requirements. The bilingual form helps students to accumulate English professional vocabulary and improve their reading ability, so as to lay a foundation for paper writing. On the other hand, it is also conducive to enhancing their ability to participate in external exchanges and cooperation.

This textbook is written by the experienced professors and scholars in pharmaceutics. The English revision is completed by Ms. Zhang Jinqiu. We would like to acknowledge the kindly support from our editorial board members and their institutes, as well as China Medical Science Press.

This textbook is suitable for undergraduate experimental teaching of Chinese Materia Medica, pharmacy, pharmaceutical engineering and other related majors.

Due to the limited capacity of authors, it is inevitable that there are some deficiencies in content arrangement and English expression. We look forward to your valuable comments and suggestions.

Authors

April 2020

目录 ┆ Contents

模块一　制剂基础性实验
Module I　Basic Experiments of Pharmaceutical Preparations

模块二　制剂评价技术

Module II　Evaluation Technologies of Pharmaceutical Preparations

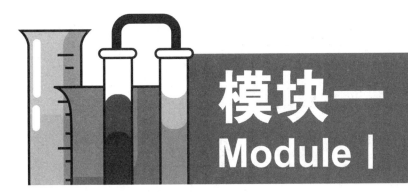

模块一
Module I

制剂基础性实验
Basic Experiments of Pharmaceutical Preparations

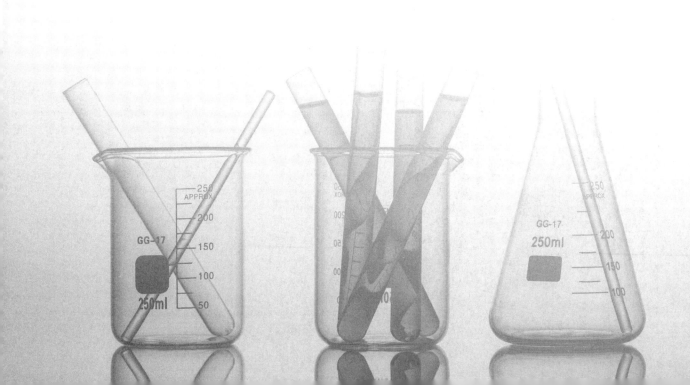

实验一 低分子溶液剂的制备

实验目的

1. **掌握** 低分子溶液剂的基本制备方法。
2. **熟悉** 不同类型低分子溶液剂的配制特点及附加剂的使用。

实验原理

低分子溶液剂系指小分子药物溶解在适宜溶剂中形成的均相液体制剂，供内服或外用。常用的溶剂有水、乙醇、甘油、丙二醇、脂肪油等，根据需要可加入助溶剂、增溶剂、抗氧剂、防腐剂、矫味剂等附加剂。低分子溶液剂包括溶液剂、芳香水剂、糖浆剂、甘油剂、酊剂、醑剂等。

溶液剂指小分子药物以分子或离子状态溶解在溶剂中形成的澄明液体制剂，其药物通常无挥发性，溶剂多为水。制备方法有溶解法、稀释法和化学反应法。

芳香水剂指芳香挥发性药物的饱和或近饱和的水溶液，多用作矫味剂或防腐剂。其制备方法因原料而异，有溶解法、稀释法、蒸馏法等，原料为化学药物时多用溶解法、稀释法制备，原料为含挥发性成分的植物药材则多用蒸馏法制备。采用分散剂分散或振摇等措施可增加油水接触面积，也可加适量增溶剂增大挥发性药物在水中的溶解度。

糖浆剂系指含有药物或芳香物质的浓蔗糖水溶液。单糖浆含糖量为85%（g/ml）或64.7%（g/g），药用糖浆含糖量应不低于45%（g/ml）。糖浆剂除另有规定外，一般是将药物用新沸过的水溶解后，加入单糖浆；如直接加入蔗糖配制，则需加水煮沸，必要时滤过，并自滤器上添加适量新沸过的水，使成处方规定量，搅匀即得。

低分子溶液剂的制备方法通常为：取处方量1/2~3/4的溶剂，加入药物搅拌溶解，必要时加热。若有液体药物，可加入混合均匀。最后自滤器上加适量的溶剂至所需量，摇匀即可。

制备低分子溶液剂的一般原则为：①溶解度大的固体药物直接溶解，溶解度小的药物应先将其溶解后再加入其他药物，可采用微粉化、加热、助溶、增溶及采用混合溶剂等措施促进溶解；②毒、剧药应先溶解，并保证溶解完全；③易氧化的药物，可加抗氧剂、金属络合剂等稳定剂及pH调节剂等；④无防腐能力的药物及溶剂，应加防腐剂；⑤含醇性液体加到水溶液中时，速度要慢，且应边加边搅拌；⑥成品应进行质量检查，合格后选用适宜洁净容器包装，并贴上标签（一般内服液体制剂用白底蓝字或白底黑字标签，外用液体制剂用白底红字或黄字标签）。

实验器材

1. **仪器** 研钵、烧杯、具塞三角瓶、玻璃漏斗、量筒、天平、电炉、滤纸、脱脂棉、玻璃棒等。

2. 材料 碘、碘化钾、滑石粉、薄荷油、聚山梨酯 80、蔗糖、蒸馏水等。

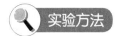 **实验方法**

（一）复方碘溶液的制备

【处方】

碘	2.5g
碘化钾	5.0g
蒸馏水	加至 50ml

【制法】取碘化钾，加蒸馏水适量，配成浓溶液，再加碘溶解，添加适量的蒸馏水至 50ml，摇匀，即得。

【性状】本品为红棕色的澄清液体；有碘的特臭。

【用途】本品内服可调节甲状腺功能，用于治疗缺碘引起的疾病的辅助治疗，如甲状腺肿大、甲状腺功能亢进等。外用可作为黏膜消毒剂。

【注意事项】

（1）碘在水中的溶解度为 1 : 2950，加碘化钾作助溶剂形成易溶性的 KI_3 络合物，增加碘在水中的溶解度，并使溶液稳定，同时减少其刺激性。

（2）为使碘能迅速溶解，需将碘化钾加少量水（1 : 1）配成浓溶液，然后加入碘溶解。

（3）碘有腐蚀性，称量时可用玻璃器皿或蜡纸，不要接触皮肤与黏膜。碘溶液为强氧化剂，应贮于密闭玻璃瓶内，不得与木塞、橡胶塞及金属接触。

（二）不同处方薄荷水的制备

【处方】

	处方 I	处方 II	处方 III
薄荷油	0.2ml	0.2ml	0.2ml
滑石粉	1.5g		
聚山梨酯 80		1.2g	1.2g
90% 乙醇			60.0ml
蒸馏水	加至 100.0ml	100.0ml	100.0ml

【制法】

（1）处方 I 用分散溶解法　取薄荷油，加滑石粉，在研钵中研匀，移至具塞三角瓶中，加入蒸馏水，加盖，振摇 10 分钟，反复过滤至滤液澄明，再由滤器上加适量蒸馏水，使成 100ml，即得。

（2）处方 II 用增溶法　取薄荷油，加聚山梨酯 80 搅匀，加入蒸馏水充分搅拌溶解，过滤至滤液澄明，再由滤器上加适量蒸馏水，使成 100ml，即得。

（3）处方 III 用增溶 - 复溶剂法　取薄荷油，加聚山梨酯 80 搅匀，在搅拌下，缓慢加入 90% 乙醇及纯化水适量溶解，过滤至滤液澄明，再由滤器上加适量纯化水制成 100ml，即得。

【性状】本品为无色透明的澄清液体，具有薄荷清香气味。

【用途】芳香调味药与祛风药，用于胃肠胀气。亦可作为分散溶媒用。

【注意事项】

（1）本品为薄荷油的饱和水溶液（约 0.05%，ml/ml），处方用量为饱和溶解度的 4 倍，配制时不能完全溶解。

（2）滑石粉为分散剂，应与薄荷油充分混匀，以利于发挥其作用，加速溶解过程。

（3）聚山梨酯 80 为增溶剂，应先与薄荷油充分混匀，再加水溶解，以利发挥增溶作用。

（三）单糖浆的制备

【处方】

蔗糖	85.0g
蒸馏水	加至 100.0ml

【制法】取蒸馏水 45ml，煮沸，加蔗糖，搅拌使溶解，趁热用脱脂棉过滤，自滤器上添加适量热蒸馏水至全量，搅匀，即得。

【性状】本品为无色至淡黄色的澄清稠厚液体，味甜。

【用途】矫味剂，助悬剂，供制备药用糖浆等。

【注意事项】蔗糖溶解后应继续煮沸，但时间不宜过长，否则蔗糖可水解为转化糖（葡萄糖和果糖），转化糖含量过高，在贮存期容易发酵，影响糖浆剂质量。

实验结果与讨论

1. **结果** 将复方碘溶液、薄荷水及单糖浆的性状检查结果记录于表 1-1。

表 1-1　复方碘溶液、薄荷水及单糖浆性状检查结果

制剂		颜色	澄明度	嗅味
复方碘溶液				
薄荷水	处方 I			
	处方 II			
	处方 III			
单糖浆				

2. **讨论** 比较不同处方薄荷水样品的性状，分析三种制备方法的特点。

思考题

1. 增加药物溶解度的方法有哪些？
2. 影响聚山梨酯 80 增溶效果的因素有哪些？
3. 增溶与助溶有何区别？
4. 配制糖浆剂时应注意哪些问题？

（韩　丽　张定堃）

Lab. 1 Preparation of Low Molecular Solutions

 Experimental Objectives

1. To master the basic preparation methods of low molecular solutions.

2. To be familiar with the preparation characteristics of different types of low molecular solutions and the use of additives.

 Experimental Principles

Low molecular solutions refer to homogeneous liquid preparation made by dissolving small molecule drugs in suitable solvent. It is for internal or external use. Commonly used solvents include water, ethanol, glycerin, propylene glycol, fat oil, etc. According to the needs, it can add hydrotropic agents, solubilizers, antioxidants, preservatives, flavoring agents and other additives. Low molecular solutions can be divided into solutions, aromatic water, syrups, glycerins, tinctures, spirits, etc.

Solutions refer to a kind of clear liquid preparation formed by dissolving small molecular drugs in the solvent in molecular or ionic state. The drugs are usually nonvolatile, and the solvent is mainly water. The preparation methods include dissolution method, dilution method and chemical reaction method.

Aromatic water refers to the saturated or nearly saturated aqueous solution of aromatic volatile drugs, which is mostly used as flavoring agents or preservatives. The preparation methods vary according to the raw materials, including dissolution method, dilution method, distillation method, etc. When the raw materials are chemical drugs, dissolution method and dilution method are often used, while when they are plant medicinal materials containing volatile components, distillation method is often adopted. It is that the measures of dispersant dispersion or shaking can increase the contact area of oil and water, as well as adding appropriate solubilizers, which are benefit for improving the solubility of volatile drugs in water.

Syrups refer to concentrated sucrose solution containing medicine or aromatic substances. The sugar content of simple syrup is 85% (g/ml) or 64.7% (g/g) , and that of medical syrup is more than 45% (g/ml). Apart from otherwise rule, syrups are generally made by dissolving the medicine in newly boiled water and adding single syrup. If it is prepared by adding sucrose directly, it needs to be boiled with water, even filtered if necessary, and adding a proper amount of newly boiling water from the filter to make it reach the prescribed amount, stir thoroughly until it is even.

The preparation method of low molecular solutions is usually as follows: Take 1/2~3/4 solvent of prescription amount, add medicine to stir and dissolve, even heat if necessary. If there is liquid medicine, it can be added and mixed evenly. Finally, add a proper amount of solvent from the filter to make it reach the prescribed amount, stir thoroughly until it is even.

The general principles for the preparation of low molecular solutions are as follows: ① Solid drugs with high solubility can be dissolved directly, while the drugs with low solubility should be dissolved first and then added to other drugs. Some measures such as micronization, heating, hydrotropy, solubilization and mixed solvents can be used to promote dissolution. ② For the toxic and drastic drugs, it should be dissolved first to ensure complete dissolution. ③ For the easily oxidized drugs, stabilizers such as antioxidant, metal complexing agent and pH regulator can be added. ④ For drugs and solvents without antiseptic capacity, it is better to add preservatives. ⑤ When the alcoholic liquid is added into the aqueous solution, the speed shall be slow, and the stirring shall be maintained. ⑥ The finished products should be checked for quality. After being qualified, they should be packed in suitable clean containers and labeled (In general, the liquid preparations for internal use are labeled with blue or black characters on white background, while those for external use are labeled with red or yellow characters on white background).

 Equipments and Materials

1. Equipments Mortar, beaker, conical flask with stopper, glass funnel, graduated cylinder, balance, electric furnace, filter paper, absorbent cotton, glass rod, etc.

2. Materials Iodine, potassium iodide, talcum powder, peppermint oil, polysorbate 80, sucrose, distilled water, etc.

 Experimental Methods

I. Preparation of Compound Iodine Solution

【Formula】

Iodine	2.5g
Potassium iodide	5.0g
Distilled water	Add to 50ml

【Procedure】Take potassium iodide, add a proper amount of distilled water, prepare a concentrated solution. Then, add iodine to dissolve, and add a proper amount of distilled water to 50ml, shake well, and then obtain.

【Description】Red brown color, clear liquid, and special odor of iodine.

【Application】Oral administration of compound iodine solution can regulate the thyroid function, and is used for the adjuvant treatment of diseases caused by iodine deficiency, such as goiter, hyperthyroidism, etc. It can also be used as a mucosal disinfectant for external use.

【Notes】

(1) The solubility of iodine in water is 1 : 2950. Potassium iodide is added as a hydrotropic agent to form a soluble KI_3 complex, which can increase the solubility of iodine in water, stabilize the solution and reduce its irritation.

(2) To make iodine dissolve rapidly, it is necessary to add a small amount of water (1 : 1) into potassium iodide to prepare a concentrated solution, and then add iodine to dissolve it.

(3) Iodine is corrosive. Glassware or wax paper can be used for weighing. Be careful not to contact skin and mucous membrane. Iodine solution is a strong oxidant and should be stored in a closed glass bottle. It should not contact with wood plug, rubber plug or metal.

II. Preparation of Peppermint Water with Different Formulas

【Formula】

	Formula I	Formula II	Formula III
Peppermint oil	0.2ml	0.2ml	0.2ml
Talcum powder	1.5g		
Polysorbate 80		1.2g	1.2g
90% Ethanol			60.0ml
Distilled water	Add to 100.0ml	100.0ml	100.0ml

【Procedure】

(1) Dispersive dissolution method is used to prepare Formula I. Take peppermint oil, add talcum powder, grind them in mortar, then transfer into a triangular flask with stopper. Add distilled water, cover it, shake for 10min, repeatedly filter until the filtrate is clear, and then add a proper amount of distilled water to make it reach 100ml.

(2) Solubilization method is used to prepare Formula II. Take peppermint oil, add polysorbate 80, and mix well. Add distilled water to fully mix and dissolve, filter until the filtrate is clear, and then add a proper amount of distilled water to the filter to make it reach 100ml.

(3) Solubilization and complex solvents method is used to prepare Formula III. Take peppermint oil, add polysorbate 80, and mix well. Under stirring, add 90% ethanol slowly and a certain amount of purified water to dissolve, filter until the filtrate is clear, and then add a certain amount of purified water to make it reach 100ml.

【Description】Colorless, transparent liquid, and mint fragrance.

【Application】Aromatic flavoring medicine and wind dispelling medicine. It can be used in the treatment of gastrointestinal inflation. It can also be used as a dispersed solvent.

【Notes】

(1) It is the saturated water solution of peppermint oil (about 0.05%, ml/ml). The prescription dosage is about 4 times of the saturated solubility. It can not be completely dissolved during preparation.

(2) Talcum powder, as a dispersant, should be fully mixed with peppermint oil to accelerate the dissolution process.

(3) Polysorbate 80 is a solubilizer, which should be fully mixed with peppermint oil, and then dissolved with water to play the solubilization role.

III. Preparation of Simple Syrup

【Formula】

Sucrose	85.0g
Distilled water	Add to 100.0ml

【Procedure】Take 45ml distilled water and boil it. Add sucrose, stir to dissolve, filter with absorbent cotton while it is hot, add proper amount of hot distilled water from the filter to the full amount, shake well, and then obtain.

【Description】Colorless to light yellow, clear and viscous liquid, and sweet taste.

【Application】Simple syrup can be used as flavoring agent and suspending agent. It is also used for the preparation of medicinal syrup.

【Notes】After the sucrose dissolves, it should continue to boil. But the time should not be too long, otherwise, the sucrose can be hydrolyzed to invert sugar (glucose and fructose). If the content of invert sugar is too high, it is easy to ferment in the storage period, which affects the quality of syrup.

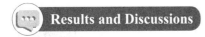 **Results and Discussions**

1. Results The examination results of the properties of compound iodine solution, peppermint water and single syrup should be recorded in the Table 1–1.

Table 1–1 The properties of compound iodine solution, peppermint water and single syrup

Preparations		Color inspection	Clarity inspection	Smelling inspection
Compound iodine solution				
Peppermint water	Formula I			
	Formula II			
	Formula III			
Simple syrup				

2. Discussions Analysis of the characteristics of three preparation methods of peppermint water.

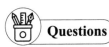 **Questions**

1. What are the ways to increase the solubility of drugs?
2. What are the factors that affect the solubilization of polysorbate 80?
3. What is the difference between solubilization and hydrotropy?
4. What should be paid attention to when preparing syrup?

实验二　高分子溶液剂的制备

实验目的

1. **掌握**　高分子化合物的溶解特性和制备高分子溶液的方法。
2. **熟悉**　高分子溶液的特点和常见的高分子材料的种类及性能。
3. **了解**　影响高分子溶液性质的因素。

实验原理

　　高分子溶液剂系指高分子化合物溶解于溶剂中制成的均相液体制剂，以水为溶剂的高分子溶液剂称为亲水性高分子溶液剂（又称亲水胶或胶浆剂），以非水溶剂制备的高分子溶液剂，称为非水性高分子溶液剂，两者均属于热力学稳定体系。高分子溶液剂具有荷电性、渗透压、黏度、聚结以及胶凝性等性质。

　　亲水性高分子溶液中的高分子物质含有大量的亲水基团，能与水形成牢固的水化膜，进而阻止分子之间的相互凝聚，使高分子溶液处于稳定状态。大量电解质或脱水剂的加入会破坏水化膜而导致高分子溶液剂发生絮凝现象。此外，高分子化合物的荷电性会通过静电斥力维持体系的稳定，带相反电荷的高分子物质的加入会因电荷中和作用产生凝结沉淀现象。

　　高分子化合物的溶解过程主要是溶胀的过程，一般包括有限溶胀和无限溶胀过程。有限溶胀是指水分子渗透进入高分子化合物结构的空隙中，与其亲水基团发生水化作用而使体积溶胀，结果使高分子空隙间充满水分子。随着溶胀过程继续，水分子降低高分子化合物分子间的作用力（范德华力），进而使化合物完全分散在水中形成高分子溶液，这一过程称为无限溶胀。制备高分子溶液剂的关键是基于高分子化合物的性质控制好有限溶胀和无限溶胀的工艺条件，如明胶溶液的制备，需要把明胶碎成小块，放于水中浸泡 3~4 小时，使其吸水溶胀，待完全溶胀后，加热搅拌形成明胶溶液。

$$\boxed{高分子材料} \xrightarrow[\text{有限溶胀}]{\text{浸泡}} \xrightarrow[\text{无限溶胀}]{\text{搅拌}} \boxed{高分子溶液}$$

　　高分子药物有胃蛋白酶、聚维酮等。常用的药用高分子材料包括天然高分子材料和合成高分子材料。前者主要有醋酸纤维素、醋酸纤维素酞酸酯、羧甲基纤维素钠、甲基纤维素、乙基纤维素、羟丙基甲基纤维素等，后者主要包括卡波姆、丙烯酸树脂、聚乙烯醇、聚维酮、乙烯－醋酸乙烯共聚物、聚乙二醇、泊洛沙姆、聚丙烯酸和聚丙烯酸钠等材料。

实验器材

1. **仪器**　托盘天平、pH 计、量筒、乳钵、玻棒、烧杯、电炉、具塞三角瓶等。
2. **材料**　胃蛋白酶、橙皮酊、稀盐酸、单糖浆、羧甲基纤维素钠（CMC-Na）、甘油、羟苯乙酯、乙醇、氯化钠、硫酸铜、蒸馏水等。

实验方法

（一）胃蛋白酶合剂的制备

【处方】

胃蛋白酶	3.0g
橙皮酊	5.0ml
稀盐酸	2.0ml
单糖浆	15.0ml
蒸馏水	加至 100ml

【制法】取稀盐酸、单糖浆混合后加蒸馏水至 90ml，摇匀，将胃蛋白酶均匀撒布在液面上，令其自然浸透膨胀，下沉后，沿同一方向轻轻搅拌使溶解，再加入橙皮酊，加水至全量，搅拌均匀，即得。

【性状】本品为微黄色高分子溶液剂，有橙皮芳香气，味酸甜。

【用途】本品为助消化药，用于因进食蛋白性食物过多及胃蛋白酶缺乏引起的消化不良症，或病后恢复期消化机能减退等症。

【注意事项】

（1）胃蛋白酶溶解时，其有限溶胀和无限溶胀过程都很快，需将其自然溶胀后再搅拌，如将之撒布于液面后立即搅拌则形成团块，给制备过程带来困难。同时应注意胃蛋白酶在温度过高（40℃左右）环境下易失活，故制备过程需严格控制温度。

（2）胃蛋白酶为一种消化酶，能使蛋白质分解为蛋白胨。因其消化力以 pH 1.5~2.5 时为最强，故常与稀盐酸配伍应用，且成品中浓度不宜过高，否则易失去活性。

（3）橙皮酊为芳香性健胃药，既是芳香矫味剂，又有一定的健胃作用。

（4）单糖浆为矫味剂，一般为蔗糖的饱和水溶液，含蔗糖 85%（g/ml），或 64.7%（g/g），最好现用现配。

（二）羧甲基纤维素钠胶浆的制备

【处方】

羧甲基纤维素钠	1.0g
甘油	12.0ml
羟苯乙酯乙醇溶液（50g/L）	0.5ml
蒸馏水	加至 40ml

【制法】取羧甲基纤维素钠分次均匀撒在 20ml 蒸馏水面，令其自然溶胀，然后稍加热并轻轻沿同一方向搅拌使溶解，加入羟苯乙酯乙醇溶液、甘油，搅匀，再加蒸馏水至全量，搅拌均匀，即得。

【性状】本品为无色透明黏稠液体。

【用途】羧甲基纤维素钠胶浆本身无治疗作用，但有一定的黏稠性。在药剂生产中常用作黏合剂、助悬剂等附加剂。

【注意事项】

（1）应先将羧甲基纤维素钠在适量冷水中充分溶胀，然后再稍加热促溶解。

（2）羧甲基纤维素钠遇阳离子型药物及碱土金属、重金属盐会发生沉淀，故不能使用季铵盐类和汞类防腐剂。

（3）甘油为润湿剂，促进 CMC-Na 溶胀过程并提高体系分散稳定性。

（三）高分子溶液剂稳定性影响因素考察

（1）取制备好的胃蛋白酶合剂，分别按体积加入 5% 氯化钠、30% 无水乙醇，观察加入前后合剂的性状变化。

（2）取制备好的羧甲基纤维素钠胶浆适量，分别按体积加入 5% 硫酸铜、30% 无水乙醇，观察加入前后胶浆剂的性状变化。

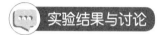 **实验结果与讨论**

1. 实验结果

（1）胃蛋白酶合剂和羧甲基纤维素钠胶浆性状检查　胃蛋白酶合剂和羧甲基纤维素钠胶浆性状检查见表 2-1。

表 2-1　胃蛋白酶合剂、羧甲基纤维素钠胶浆检查结果

制剂	颜色	外观	嗅味
胃蛋白酶合剂			
羧甲基纤维素钠胶浆			

（2）胃蛋白酶合剂和羧甲基纤维素钠胶浆 pH 测定（表 2-2）。

表 2-2　胃蛋白酶合剂、羧甲基纤维素钠胶浆 pH 测定结果

制剂	pH
胃蛋白酶合剂	
羧甲基纤维素钠胶浆	

（3）高分子溶液剂稳定性影响因素考察（表 2-3）。

表 2-3　高分子溶液剂稳定性影响因素考察结果

制剂	不同影响因素下性状变化		
	5% 氯化钠	5% 硫酸铜	30% 无水乙醇
胃蛋白酶合剂		/	
羧甲基纤维素钠胶浆	/		

2. 讨论

试分析氯化钠、硫酸铜、无水乙醇对胃蛋白酶合剂及羧甲基纤维素钠胶浆稳定性的影响。

思考题

1. 以胃蛋白酶合剂制备过程说明高分子化合物的溶解过程。
2. 导致高分子溶液聚结的因素有哪些？
3. 高分子溶液剂和溶胶剂在渗透压方面有何差别？

（邹俊波）

Lab. 2 Preparation of Polymer Solution

 Experimental Objectives

1. To master the dissolution characteristics of polymer compounds and the method of preparing polymer solution.

2. To be familiar with the characteristics of polymer solution and the types and properties of common polymer materials.

3. To understand the factors affecting the properties of polymer solution.

 Experimental Principles

Polymer solution refers to homogeneous liquid preparation made by dissolving polymer compound in solvent. Polymer solution dissolved in water is called hydrophilic polymer solution (also known as hydrophilic mucilage or mucilage) while those prepared with non-aqueous solvent is called non-aqueous polymer solution, both of which belong to thermodynamically stable system. The properties of polymer solution include charge, osmotic pressure, viscosity, coalescence and gelling.

The polymer substances in the hydrophilic polymer solution contains a large number of hydrophilic groups, which can form a solid hydration film with water to prevent the condensation between molecules and keep the polymer solution in a stable state. The hydration film destroyed by addition of a large number of electrolytes or dehydrating agents would lead to the flocculation of polymer solution. In addition, the charging property of polymer compounds will maintain the stability of the system through electrostatic repulsion, and the addition of polymer substances with opposite charge will cause condensation and precipitation due to charge neutralization.

Swelling process including limited swelling and infinite swelling is the main stage in dissolution process of polymer compounds. In limited swelling stage, water molecules infiltrate into the voids of polymer compounds and are hydrated with hydrophilic groups, which result in volume swelling and water molecules filled between polymer voids. As the swelling process continues, the intermolecular force (van der Waals force) of polymer compounds is reduced by water and completely disperse in the solvent to form polymer solution, which is called infinite swelling. The key to the preparation of polymer solution is to control the process conditions of limited swelling and infinite swelling based on the properties of polymer compounds. Take the preparation of gelatin solution for example, gelatin needs to be broken into small pieces, then absorbs water and swells by soaking in water for 3~4 hours when the solution is heated and stirred to form a gelatin solution.

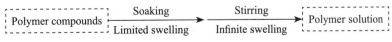

Pepsin and povidone etc. are common polymer drugs. Commonly used medicinal polymer materials include natural and synthetic polymer materials. The former mainly includes cellulose acetate, cellulose acetate phthalate, carboxymethylcellulose sodium, methyl cellulose, ethyl cellulose, hydroxypropyl methyl cellulose and so on. The latter mainly includes carbomer, acrylic resin, polyvinyl alcohol, povidone, ethylene-vinyl acetate copolymer, polyethylene glycol, poloxamer, polyacrylic acid and sodium polyacrylate, etc.

 Equipments and Materials

1. Equipments   Pallet balance, pH meter, graduated cylinder, morta, glass rod, beaker, electric furnace, conical flask with stopper, etc.

2. Materials   Pepsin, flavedo tincture, diluted hydrochloric acid, syrupus simplex, carboxymethylcellulose sodium (CMC-Na), glycerol, hydroxyphenylethyl ester, ethanol, sodium chloride, copper sulfate, distilled water, etc.

 Experimental Methods

Ⅰ. Preparation of Pepsin Mixture

【Formula】

Pepsin	3.0g
Flavedo tincture	5.0ml
Diluted hydrochloric acid	2.0ml
Syrupus simplex	15.0ml
Distilled water	Add to 100ml

【Procedure】Pipet diluted hydrochloric acid and syrupus simplex, add distilled water to 90ml, and shake well, spread pepsin evenly on the liquid surface, make it soak and expand naturally. Gently stir along the same direction to dissolve after sinking, then add flavedo tincture, add water to full amount, stir thoroughly until it is even.

【Description】Pepsin mixture is yellowish in color. It has a slightly characteristic odor of flavedo aroma which taste sweet and sour.

【Application】Pepsin mixture is a drug promoting ingestion, used for diseases such as eating too much protein food and pepsin indigestion, or digestive dysfunction in the recovery period after the disease.

【Notes】

(1) The limited swelling and infinite swelling stage when pepsin dissolves are very fast, stir only after it has swollen naturally. If it is spread on the liquid surface and stirred immediately, conglomeration would be formed, which brings difficulties to the preparation process. Attention should be paid that pepsin is easy to be inactivated when the temperature is too high (about 40℃), so the temperature should be strictly controlled in the preparation process.

(2) Pepsin is a digestive enzyme that can decompose protein into peptone of which the strongest digestibility at pH 1.5~2.5, it is often used in combination with diluted hydrochloric acid. The concentration of pepsin in medicament should not be too high, or its activity would be influenced significantly.

(3) Flavedo tincture is an aromatic stomachic which serves not only an aromatic flavor agent, but also has a certain stomach-invigorating effect.

(4) Syrupus simplex, as corrigentis, generally a saturated aqueous solution of sucrose, containing 85% (g/ml) or 64.7% (g/g) sucrose, should be prepared when needed.

II. Preparation of Carboxymethylcellulose Sodium Mucilage

【Formula】

Carboxymethyl cellulose sodium	1.0g
Glycerol	12.0ml
Hydroxyphenylethyl ester ethanol solution (50g/L)	0.5ml
Distilled water	Add to 40ml

【Procedure】Gradually sprinkle carboxymethylcellulose sodium evenly into 20ml distilled water to make it naturally swollen, then slightly heat and gently stir in the same direction to dissolve, add hydroxyphenylethyl ester ethanol solution and glycerol, stir well then add distilled water to full amount, stir thoroughly until it is even.

【Description】Colorless, transparent, and viscous liquid.

【Application】Carboxymethyl cellulose sodium mucilage itself has no therapeutic effect, but has a certain viscosity. It is often used as adhesive, suspending agent and other additives in pharmaceutical production.

【Notes】

(1) Carboxymethyl cellulose sodium should be fully swollen in moderate amounts of cold water, and then slightly heated to promote dissolution.

(2) Carboxymethyl cellulose sodium will precipitate in the presence of cationic drugs, alkaline earth metals and heavy metallic salts. Preservatives such as quaternary ammonium salts and mercury cannot be used.

(3) Glycerol is used as wetting agent to promote the swelling process of carboxymethyl cellulose sodium and improve the dispersion stability of the system.

III. Investigation on the Factors Affecting the Stability of Polymer Solution

(1) Pipet pepsin mixture prepared above, add 5% sodium chloride and 30% anhydrous ethanol respectively according to volume, please observe the changes of properties of the mixture before and after adding.

(2) Pipet carboxymethylcellulose sodium mucilage prepared above, add 5% copper sulfate and 30% anhydrous ethanol by volume, respectively. Please observe the changes of the properties of the mucilage before and after adding.

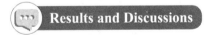 **Results and Discussions**

1. Results

(1) Examination of the properties of pepsin mixture and carboxymethylcellulose sodium mucilage. The properties of pepsin mixture and carboxymethylcellulose sodium mucilage should be recorded in the Table 2-1.

Table 2-1　The properties of pepsin mixture and carboxymethylcellulose sodium mucilage

Preparations	Color inspection	Appearance inspection	Smelling inspection
Pepsin mixture			
Carboxymethylcellulose sodium mucilage			

(2) Determination of pH of pepsin mixture and carboxymethylcellulose sodium mucilage (Table 2–2).

Table 2–2   pH value of pepsin mixture and carboxymethylcellulose sodium mucilage

Preparations	pH value
Pepsin mixture	
Carboxymethylcellulose sodium mucilage	

(3) Investigation on the factors affecting the stability of polymer solution (Table 2–3).

Table 2–3   Results of investigation on the factors affecting the stability of polymer solution

Preparations	Appearance changes under different affecting factors		
	5% Sodium chloride	5% Copper sulfate	30% Anhydrous ethanol
Pepsin mixture		/	
Carboxymethylcellulose sodium mucilage	/		

2. Discussions　　Try to analyze the effects of sodium chloride, copper sulfate and anhydrous ethanol on the stability of pepsin mixture and carboxymethylcellulose sodium mucilage.

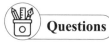 **Questions**

1. Take the preparation process of pepsin mixture for example, try to illustrate the dissolution process of polymer compounds.

2. What are the factors that lead to the coalescence of polymer solution?

3. What is the difference in osmotic pressure between polymer solution and mucilage?

实验三　乳剂的制备及乳剂类型的鉴别

PPT

 实验目的

1. **掌握**　乳剂的一般制备方法。
2. **熟悉**　乳剂类型的鉴别方法及影响乳剂稳定性的因素。

实验原理

　　两种互不混溶的液体经乳化而形成的非均相分散体系称为乳剂（也称乳浊液）。分散的液滴称为分散相、内相或不连续相，一般直径在 0.1~100μm；包在液滴外面的液相称为分散介质、外相或连续相。乳剂分为水包油型（O/W）和油包水型（W/O），常采用稀释法和染色法鉴别。

　　乳剂处方中除分散相和分散介质外，还需加入乳化剂。乳化剂一方面降低了油水两相界面张力，使乳剂容易形成；另一方面，乳化剂可在分散液滴表面形成单分子膜、多分子膜或固体微粒膜等界面膜，防止液滴相遇时发生合并，增加乳剂的稳定性。常用的乳化剂为表面活性剂。

　　制备少量乳剂时，可采用在乳钵中研磨或瓶中振摇等方法；大量生产可采用搅拌机、胶体磨和乳匀机等设备进行制备。一般可根据 HLB 值选择乳化剂。当一种乳化剂难以达到乳化要求时，常将两种或两种以上的乳化剂混合使用。混合乳化剂的 HLB 值可按下式计算：

$$HLB_{混合} = \frac{HLB_1 \cdot W_1 + HLB_2 \cdot W_2 + \cdots + HLB_n \cdot W_n}{W_1 + W_2 + \cdots + W_n}$$

式中，HLB_1，HLB_2，$\cdots$，HLB_n 为各个乳化剂的 HLB 值；W_1，W_2，$\cdots$，W_n 为各个乳化剂的质量分数或质量。

实验器材

1. **仪器**　研钵、烧杯、量筒、具塞试剂瓶、天平、试管、载玻片、称量纸、玻璃棒等。
2. **材料**　液状石蜡、阿拉伯胶、西黄蓍胶、羟苯乙酯、无水乙醇、蒸馏水、氢氧化钙、花生油、苏丹红、亚甲蓝等。

实验方法

（一）液状石蜡乳的制备

【处方】

液状石蜡	12.0ml
阿拉伯胶	4.0g

西黄蓍胶	0.5g
羟苯乙酯乙醇溶液（5%）	0.1ml
蒸馏水	加至 30ml

【制法】将阿拉伯胶粉与西黄蓍胶粉置于干燥的研钵中，加入液状石蜡，稍加研磨，使胶粉混合均匀后加蒸馏水 8ml，不断研磨至形成稠厚的乳状液，即初乳。再加蒸馏水、羟苯乙酯乙醇溶液，研匀，即得。

【性状】本品为乳白色黏稠液体。

【用途】轻泻剂。用于治疗便秘，特别适合于高血压、动脉瘤、疝气、痔疮及手术后便秘的病人，可以减轻排便的痛苦。

【注意事项】

（1）5% 羟苯乙酯乙醇溶液的配制　将 5g 羟苯乙酯溶于 100ml 无水乙醇中，使其完全溶解，即得。

（2）液状石蜡乳的制备　采用的是干胶法，制备初乳时应注意油、水、乳化剂的比例，并注意用力、同向、持续研磨。

（二）石灰搽剂的制备

【处方】

花生油	10ml
氢氧化钙饱和水溶液	10ml

【制法】量取花生油和氢氧化钙饱和水溶液各 10ml，置于具塞试剂瓶中，加塞，用力振摇至乳剂形成，即得。

【性状】本品为乳白色黏稠油状液体。

【用途】用于治疗轻度烫伤。具有收敛、保护、润滑、止痛等作用。

【注意事项】

（1）石灰搽剂的制备方法是新生皂法。振摇时间要充分。

（2）氢氧化钙饱和水溶液的制备　取氢氧化钙 0.2g 加至 50ml 蒸馏水中，水浴加热并充分搅拌后，冷却至室温，滤纸过滤，即得。

（三）乳剂类型的鉴别

（1）稀释法　取 2 支试管，分别加入液状石蜡乳和石灰搽剂各 1ml，再加入蒸馏水约 5ml，振摇并翻转数次，观察混合情况，判断乳剂所属类型（能与水均匀混合者为 O/W 型，反之则为 W/O 型乳剂）。

（2）染色法　将液状石蜡乳和石灰搽剂分别涂在载玻片上，用苏丹红溶液（油溶性染料）和亚甲蓝溶液（水溶液性染料）各染色一次，肉眼观察，判断乳剂所属类型（苏丹红均匀分散者为 W/O 型乳剂，亚甲蓝均匀分散者为 O/W 型乳剂）。

【注意事项】

（1）亚甲蓝溶液的配制　将 5g 亚甲蓝溶于 100ml 蒸馏水中，使其完全溶解，即得。

（2）苏丹红溶液的配制　将 0.02g 苏丹红溶于 60ml 无水乙醇中，使其完全溶解加水稀释至 100ml，即得。

实验结果与讨论

1. 实验结果

（1）液状石蜡乳、石灰搽剂性状检查　将液状石蜡乳、石灰搽剂性状检查结果填于表 3-1。

表 3-1　液状石蜡乳、石灰搽剂检查结果

制剂	颜色	外观	嗅味
液状石蜡乳			
石灰搽剂			

（2）液状石蜡乳、石灰搽剂类型鉴别结果填于表 3-2。

表 3-2　液状石蜡乳、石灰搽剂类型鉴别结果

制剂	水稀释结果	苏丹红染色	亚甲蓝染色	乳剂类型
液状石蜡乳				
石灰搽剂				

2. 讨论

（1）分析液状石蜡乳的处方并说明各成分的作用。

（2）石灰搽剂的乳化剂是什么？属于何种类型的乳剂？

思考题

1. 如何判断乳剂的类型？

2. 影响乳剂稳定性的因素有哪些？

3. 干胶法和湿胶法有何区别？

（李　文）

Lab. 3 Preparation and Type Identification of Emulsions

 Experimental Objectives

1. To master the general preparation methods of emulsions.
2. To be familiar with the judgment methods of emulsion types and the influence factors of emulsion stability.

 Experimental Principles

Two immiscible liquids are emulsified to form a non-homogeneous dispersion system called emulsions. Dispersed droplets can be called dispersed phase, internal phase or discontinuous phase, the general diameter is among 0.1μm to 100μm. Outside the liquid droplets is known as dispersion medium, external phase or continuous phase. Emulsions can be divided into water in oil type(O/W) and oil in water type (W/O), often distinguished by dilution method and staining method.

In addition to the dispersed phase and dispersion medium, the emulsifier is also added. On the one hand, emulsions can be easily formed because the emulsifier can reduce the interfacial tension between oil and water. On the other hand, the emulsifier may be due to a interfacial film formed on the surface of the scattered droplets which can prevent the merger occuring and increase stability when droplets encounter, such as monolayer number, multicellular membrane, solid powder, etc. A variety of surface active agents are commonly used as emulsifier.

To prepare a little amount of emulsions, methods can be used such as grinding in the bowl or shaking in the bottle, etc. If a mass of emulsions should be produced, mixer, colloid mill and homogenization machine can be used. Generally, the emulsifier can be chosen according to *HLB* value. As only one kind of emulsifier can not achieve such a request, two or more emulsifiers are often mixed. Mixed emulsifiers of HLB value can be calculated as follows:

$$HLB_{mix} = \frac{HLB_1 \cdot W_1 + HLB_2 \cdot W_2 + \cdots + HLB_n \cdot W_n}{W_1 + W_2 + \cdots + W_n}$$

Where, HLB_1, HLB_2, ..., HLB_n are every emulsifier's *HLB*; W_1, W_2, ..., W_n are the weight of emulsifier.

 Equipments and Materials

1. Equipments Mortar, beaker, cylinder, reagent bottle with a stopper, balance, test tube, glass slide, weighing paper, glass rod, etc.

2. Materials Liquid paraffin, acacia, tragacanth, ethylparaben, anhydrous ethanol , distilled water, calcium hydroxide, peanut oil, Sudan, methylene blue, etc.

Experimental Methods

I. Preparation of Liquid Paraffin Emulsion

【Formula】

Liquid paraffin	12.0ml
Acacia	4.0g
Tragacanth	0.5g
Ethylparaben alcohol solution(5%)	0.1ml
Distilled water	Add to 30ml

【Procedure】Combine the acacia and tragacanth in a dry mortar and mix, then add liquid paraffin and triturate until the two gums dispersed completely. Add 8ml distill water and triturate continuously until a dense primary emulsion is formed. Add residuary distilled water and ethylparaben alcohol solution with constant trituration. Keep grinding until the emulsion is formed.

【Description】The product is a kind of milk white viscous liquid.

【Application】Aperient. Medication for constipation. Especially for constipation caused by hypertension, aneurysms, hernias, surgical patients with hemorrhoids. It can reduce the pain of defecation.

【Notes】

(1) Preparation of 5% ethylparaben alcohol solution: Put 5g ethylparaben in 100ml anhydrous ethanol and dissolve completely.

(2) Liquid paraffin emulsion is made by emulsifier-in-oil method. The ratio of oil, water and emulsifier should be noteworthy during the preparation of primary emulsion. Pay attention to grinding vigorously and continuously in the same direction.

II. Preparation of Lime Liniment

【Formula】

Peanut oil	10ml
Calcium hydroxide saturated solution	10ml

【Procedure】Measure 10ml peanut oil and calcium hydroxide saturated solution separately. Put them in a reagent bottle with a stopper and seal, then shake vigorously until the emulsion is formed.

【Description】The product is a kind of milk white viscous oily liquid.

【Application】Use for slight burns. It possesses the function of convergence, protection, lubrication and alleviating pain.

【Notes】

(1) The emulsion of lime liniment is a nascent calcium soap generated from reaction between calcium hydroxide solution and free fatty acid in peanut oil. The shaking force should be strong for enough time.

(2) Preparation of calcium hydroxide saturated solution: Put 0.2g calcium hydroxide in 50ml distilled water, then heat in water bath and stir thoroughly. After reaction is finished, the product is cooled to room temperature before filter.

III. Identification of Emulsion's Type

(1) Dilution method: Take two tubes, add 1ml liquid paraffin and lime liniment separately, then add distilled water about 5ml. Shake and turnover several times to observe the mixing status. At last, determine the type of emulsions (O/W type could mix with water, otherwise W/O type).

(2) Staining method: Put liquid paraffin and lime liniment on the glass slide separately. Use Sudan solution (oil-soluble dye) and methylene blue solution (water-soluble dye) staining one time separately. Then observe by eyes and judge the type of emulsions (Sudan could be well dispersed in W/O type, Methylene blue could be well dispersed in O/W type).

【Notes】

(1) Preparation of methylene blue solution: Put 5g Methylene blue in 100ml distilled water and dissolve completely.

(2) Preparation of Sudan: Put 0.02g Sudan in 60ml anhydrous ethanol and dissolve completely, then add distilled water to 100ml.

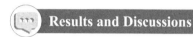 **Results and Discussions**

1. Results

(1) The property tests of liquid paraffin emulsion and lime liniment. Filling the results in the Table 3-1 below.

Table 3-1   **The test results of liquid paraffin emulsion and lime liniment**

Preparation	Color	Appearance	Odor
Liquid paraffin emulsion			
Lime liniment			

(2) The results of the type identification of liquid paraffin emulsion and lime liniment (Table 3-2).

Table 3-2   **The results of the type identification of liquid paraffin emulsion and lime liniment**

Preparation	Result of water dilution	Sudan dyeing	Methylene blue dyeing	Type of the emulsions
Liquid paraffin emulsion				
Lime liniment				

2. Discussions

(1) Try to analyze the formula of liquid paraffin emulsion and explain the function of each component.

(2) What is the emulsifier of lime liniment? Which type of emulsion is it?

 Questions

1. How to determine the type of the emulsions?

2. What are the factors affecting the stability of emulsifier?

3. What is the difference between emulsifier-in-oil method and emulsifier-in-water method?

实验四 混悬剂的制备及稳定剂的选择

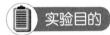 **实验目的**

1. **掌握** 混悬剂的一般制备方法及稳定剂的选择方法。
2. **熟悉** 助悬剂、润湿剂、絮凝剂及反絮凝剂在混悬剂中的应用。

实验原理

混悬剂是指难溶性固体药物以细小的微粒分散在液体溶媒中形成的非均相液体制剂，药物微粒一般在 0.5~10μm 之间。混悬剂的分散介质多为水，也可用植物油。大多数的混悬剂是液体制剂，若按照混悬剂的要求，将药物用适宜方法制成粉末状或颗粒状制剂，使用时加水即迅速分散成混悬剂，则称为干混悬剂。合剂、搽剂、洗剂、注射剂、滴眼剂、气雾剂等剂型都有混悬的分散状态。

优良的混悬剂应符合如下要求：粒子细腻、分散均匀、不结块；粒子的沉降速度慢、沉降容积比（*F*）大；颗粒沉降后，经振摇易再分散，以保证分剂量的准确性；混悬剂应具有一定黏度；外用混悬剂应容易涂布。

物理稳定性是混悬剂存在的主要问题之一。混悬剂中药物微粒的分散度大，使混悬剂具有较高的表面自由能而处于不稳定状态。疏水性药物的混悬剂比亲水性药物存在更大的稳定性问题。混悬剂中的微粒受重力作用产生沉降，其沉降速度遵循 Stock's 定律，如式（4-1）所示：

$$V = \frac{2r^2(\rho_1 - \rho_2)g}{9\eta} \qquad (4-1)$$

式中，*V* 为微粒沉降速度（cm/s）；*r* 为微粒半径（cm）；ρ_1、ρ_2 分别为微粒和分散介质的密度（g/ml）；g 为重力加速度（cm/s²）；*η* 为分散介质的黏度（mPa·s）。

从式（4-1）可看出：混悬液中微粒沉降速度与微粒半径平方、微粒与分散介质的密度差成正比；与分散介质的黏度成反比。混悬剂微粒沉降速度愈大，动力学稳定性愈小。增加混悬剂动力稳定性的主要方法有：①减小微粒的半径；②降低微粒与分散介质的密度差；③增加分散介质的黏度。因此，在制备混悬剂时，将药物粉碎成一定细度的微粒、加入助悬剂、选择适宜的分散介质等手段都能提高混悬剂的物理稳定性。

混悬剂的稳定剂一般有三类：助悬剂、润湿剂、絮凝剂与反絮凝剂。

混悬剂的配制方法有分散法（如研磨粉碎）和凝聚法（物理凝聚法和化学凝聚法）两种，其中分散法较为常用。

混悬剂的稳定性直接决定其质量好坏，混悬剂常见的稳定性研究方法包括：微粒大小的测定、沉降速度的测定、沉降容积比的测定、絮凝度的测定、重新分散实验、ξ电位的测定、流变学测定。

混悬剂的成品在包装时，容器不宜盛装太满，应预留适当空间便于用前摇匀。标签上应注明"用前摇匀"字样。为安全起见，剧、毒药及剂量小的药物不宜制成混悬剂。

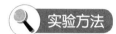

实验器材

1. **仪器** 天平、研钵、具塞量筒、玻璃棒、烧杯、称量纸、药匙、标签纸等。
2. **材料** 炉甘石、氧化锌、甘油、羧甲基纤维素钠、聚山梨酯80、枸橼酸钠、三氯化铝、沉降硫黄、硫酸锌、樟脑、乙醇、新洁尔灭、蒸馏水等。

实验方法

（一）不同处方炉甘石洗剂的制备
【处方】

	处方Ⅰ	处方Ⅱ	处方Ⅲ	处方Ⅳ	处方Ⅴ
炉甘石	4g	4g	4g	4g	4g
氧化锌	4g	4g	4g	4g	4g
甘油	5ml	5ml	5ml	5ml	5ml
羧甲基纤维素钠	0.25g				
聚山梨酯80		1.0ml			
枸橼酸钠			0.25g		
三氯化铝				0.1g	
蒸馏水	加至50ml	50ml	50ml	50ml	50ml

【制法】

（1）炉甘石、氧化锌过120目筛；羧甲基纤维素钠加水25ml，溶胀，制成胶浆；聚山梨酯80加水25ml混匀；枸橼酸钠加水25ml溶解；三氯化铝加水25ml溶解。

（2）采用加液研磨法制备。先将炉甘石和氧化锌置研钵中，加甘油研磨至糊状，再按上述不同处方加入其他成分，研磨均匀后倒出，研钵用10ml蒸馏水分次冲洗，与药液合并后加蒸馏水至50ml，即得。

【性状】本品为粉红色混悬液，放置有沉淀，经振摇后，仍应成为均匀的混悬液。

【用途】具有保护皮肤、收敛、消炎和止痒作用，用于潮红、肿胀、灼热、瘙痒而无渗出的急性皮炎、湿疹、荨麻疹、丘疹、夏季皮炎、日晒伤等皮肤病。

【注意事项】

（1）炉甘石、氧化锌均为水中不溶的亲水性药物，可被水润湿，先加入适量甘油研磨成糊状，使粉末周围形成水的保护膜，可防止颗粒聚集，振摇时易悬浮。

（2）炉甘石洗剂中的炉甘石和氧化锌带负电，加入少量三氯化铝中和部分电荷，使炉甘石和氧化锌絮凝沉降，从而防止结块，改善分散性。

（二）复方硫磺洗剂的制备
【处方】

沉降硫黄	3g
硫酸锌溶液	25ml
樟脑醑	25ml
甘油	5ml
5%新洁尔灭溶液	4ml
蒸馏水	加至100ml

【制法】取沉降硫黄置于乳钵中，加甘油研匀。再加新洁尔灭溶液研成糊状后，缓慢加入硫

酸锌溶液，研磨均匀。以细流方式慢慢加入樟脑醑并急速研磨（或搅拌），随加随研至呈均匀混悬状，再加蒸馏水至 100ml，搅匀，即得。

【性状】本品为黄色混悬液，有硫黄、樟脑的特臭。

【用途】保护皮肤、抑制皮脂分泌、轻度杀菌与收敛。用于皮脂溢出症、痤疮、疥疮等。

【注意事项】

（1）沉降硫黄为质轻的疏水性药物，加甘油可使硫黄表面亲水，且又可增强洗剂的稠度，有利于硫黄在混悬剂中均匀分散。

（2）新洁尔灭为阳离子型表面活性剂，可降低硫黄与水的界面张力，起润湿剂的作用，使硫黄均匀分散，增强药效。

（3）樟脑醑是樟脑的 10% 醇溶液，加入时应急速搅拌或研磨，以免樟脑因溶剂改变而析出大颗粒。

（4）硫酸锌溶液的制备　称取硫酸锌 3g，溶于 25ml 水中，摇匀即得。

（三）混悬液沉降容积比的测定及重新分散性考察

【沉降容积比的测定】将不同处方炉甘石洗剂分别置 100ml 具塞量筒中，密塞，振摇 1 分钟，记录初始高度 H_0 后静置并计时，分别在 5、15、30、60、90、120 分钟记录沉降物的高度 H_u，填入表 4-1，计算沉降容积比（F）。注意具塞量筒的大小、粗细尽量一致。

【重新分散实验】将不同处方炉甘石洗剂静置一段时间（一周或根据实际情况而定），将具塞量筒倒置翻转（一反一正为一次），记录试管底部的沉降物重新分散所需要的次数，填入表 4-2 中。如试管底部沉淀物始终未分散，以"结饼"结果记入。试管底部沉淀物重新分散所需次数越少，则混悬剂的重新分散性越好。

实验结果与讨论

1. 结果

（1）沉降曲线的绘制　根据表 4-1 数据，以沉降容积比 F（H_u/H_0）为纵坐标，时间 t 为横坐标，绘制沉降曲线。

表 4-1　沉降容积比测定结果

时间 /min	炉甘石洗剂									
	处方 I		处方 II		处方 III		处方 IV		处方 V	
	H_u	F	H_u	F	H_u	F	H_u	F	H_u	F
5										
15										
30										
60										
90										
120										

25

（2）重新分散实验　将各试管底部沉降物重新分散所需要的次数，填入表 4-2 中。

表 4-2　重新分散次数

处方	炉甘石洗剂				
	处方 I	处方 II	处方 III	处方IV	处方 V
翻转次数					

2. 讨论

（1）试分析炉甘石洗剂中各稳定剂的作用。

（2）炉甘石洗剂和复方硫磺洗剂，两者在制备方法上有何区别？

思考题

1. 根据 Stock's 定律并结合处方，谈谈影响混悬剂稳定性的主要因素有哪些？

2. 优良的混悬剂应达到哪些要求？

3. 硫黄有升华硫、精制硫和沉降硫等，在复方硫磺洗剂中，为何选用沉降硫？

（储晓琴）

Lab. 4 Preparation of Suspension and Selection of Stabilizers

 Experimental Objectives

1. To master the general preparation methods of suspensions and the selection of stabilizers.

2. To be familiar with the application of suspending agents, wetting agents, flocculants and deflocculants in suspension.

 Experimental Principles

Suspension refers to heterogeneous liquid preparation formed by the dispersion of insoluble solid drugs in the liquid solvent with small particles, and the drug particles generally range from 0.5 to 10μm. The dispersion medium of the suspension is mostly water and plant oil as well. Most of the suspensions are liquid preparations. There is also dry suspension, which can be quickly dispensed into a liquid when adding water with an appearance like powder or granule. Drugs can also be suspended in other formulations such as mixtures, liniments, lotions, injections, eye drops, aerosols, etc.

Good suspensions should meet the following requirements: fine particles evenly dispersed and non-packed; slow sedimentation rates and large sedimentation volume ratio of the particles; good redispersibility by shaking after sedimentation to ensure the accuracy of the dosage; possessing certain viscosity; and character of easily spread for external use.

Physical stability is one of the main problems of suspensions. The large dispersity of the drug particles in the suspension makes the system in an unstable state with high surface free energy, which is more critical for suspensions loading hydrophobic drugs than hydrophilic ones. The particles in the suspension can be settled due to gravity, and the sedimentation rate of the particles follows Stock's law, as shown in the following formula:

$$V = \frac{2r^2 (\rho_1 - \rho_2) g}{9\eta} \qquad (4-1)$$

In the formula, V is the particle settling rate (cm/s); r is the particle radius (cm); ρ_1 and ρ_2 are the density of the particles and the dispersion medium, respectively (g/ml); g is the gravitational acceleration (cm/s^2); η is the viscosity of the dispersion medium (mPa·s).

It can be seen from the above formula that the settling rate of the particles in the suspension is proportional to the square of the particle radius and the density difference between the particles and the dispersion medium, while inversely proportional to the viscosity of the medium. The greater the sedimentation rate of the solid particles, the lower the dynamic stability of the suspensions. The main methods to increase the dynamic stability of suspensions are as follows: ① reduce the radius of the particles; ② reduce the density difference between the particles and the dispersion medium; ③ increase the viscosity of the dispersion medium. Therefore, when preparing a suspension, the physical stability of

27

the suspension can be improved by crushing the drug into fine particles, adding suspending agent, and selecting a suitable dispersion medium.

There are three types of stabilizers for suspension: suspending agents, wetting agents, flocculants and deflocculating agents.

The preparation methods of suspension include dispersing method (such as grinding) and agglomeration method (physical agglomeration method and chemical agglomeration method). Among them, the dispersing method is more commonly used.

The stability of a suspension directly determines its quality. Common stability research for suspensions include: the determination of particle size, sedimentation rate, sedimentation volume ratio, flocculation degree, re-dispersion, ξ potential and rheology.

When the finished suspension product is packaged, the container should not be too full, and appropriate space should be reserved for shaking before use. The label should indicate "shake well before use". Acute, poison, and low-dose drugs should not be made into suspensions for reasons of safety.

 Equipments and Materials

1. Equipments Counter balance, mortar, measuring cylinder with stopper, glass rod, beaker, weighing paper, medicine spoon, label paper, etc.

2. Materials Calamine, zinc oxide, glycerin, sodium carboxyl methyl cellulose, polysorbate 80, sodium citrate, aluminum chloride, precipitated sulfur, zinc sulfate, camphor, ethanol, benzalkonium bromide, distilled water, etc.

 Experimental Methods

I. Preparation of Calamine Lotion in Different Formulas
【Formula】

	I	II	III	IV	V
Calamine	4g	4g	4g	4g	4g
Zinc oxide	4g	4g	4g	4g	4g
Glycerin	5ml	5ml	5ml	5ml	5ml
Sodium carboxyl methyl cellulose	0.25g				
Polysorbate 80		1.0ml			
Sodium citrate			0.25g		
Aluminum chloride				0.1g	
Distilled water	Add to 50ml	50ml	50ml	50ml	50ml

【Procedure】

(1) Calamine and zinc oxide are passed through a 120 mesh sieve. Add 25ml water to sodium carboxyl methyl cellulose, swelled and made into mucilage. Add 25ml of water to mix polysorbate 80. Sodium citrate and Aluminum chloride is dissolved in 25ml of water, respectively.

(2) All of the five prescriptions above are prepared by the method of liquid grinding. Firstly, put

calamine and zinc oxide in mortar, grind them into plaster with glycerin. Secondly, add other components according to the prescription, grind evenly and pour it out. And then wash the mortar with 10ml distilled water for several times; finally add distilled water after combining with the medicine solution to 50ml.

【Description】Calamine lotion is pink suspension. It has precipitation after standing, and it should still become a homogeneous suspension after shaking.

【Application】Calamine lotion has the functions of protecting the skin, astringency, anti-inflammatory and antipruritic, which is used for skin diseases such as flushing, swelling, burning, itching without exudation in acute dermatitis, eczema, urticaria, papule, summer dermatitis, sunburn, etc.

【Notes】

(1) Both calamine and zinc oxide are insoluble hydrophilic drugs in water, which can be wet by water. Add an appropriate amount of glycerin to grind into a paste, so that a protective film of water is formed around the powder, which can prevent particles from gathering and be easy to suspend when shaking.

(2) Calamine and zinc oxide in calamine lotion are negatively charged. A small amount of aluminum chloride is added to neutralize part of the charge, which makes calamine and zinc oxide flocculate and settle, thereby preventing agglomeration and improving dispersion.

II. Preparation of Compound Sulfur Lotion

【Formula】

Precipitated sulfur	3g
Zinc sulfate solution	25ml
Camphor tincture	25ml
Glycerin	5ml
5% Benzalkonium bromide	4ml
Distilled water	Add to 100ml

【Procedure】Put the precipitated sulfur and glycerin in mortar and grind it evenly. Then add the benzalkonium bromide solution to grind into a paste, slowly add zinc sulfate solution and grind evenly. Slowly add camphor tincture in a thin flow way and quickly grind (or stir) it until it is evenly suspended, finally add distilled water to 100ml and stir.

【Description】Compound sulfur lotion is yellow suspension with the characteristic odor of sulfur and camphor.

【Application】Compound sulfur lotion has the functions of protecting the skin, inhibiting sebum secretion, mild sterilization and convergence, which is used for seborrhea, acne, scabies, etc.

【Notes】

(1) Precipitated sulfur is a light-weight hydrophobic drug. Adding glycerin can make the surface of sulfur hydrophilic and enhance the consistency of lotion, which is beneficial to the uniform dispersion of sulfur in the suspension.

(2) Benzalkonium bromide is a cationic surfactant, which can reduce the interfacial tension between sulfur and water, and acts as a wetting agent to uniformly disperse sulfur and enhance the efficacy.

(3) Camphor tincture is a 10% alcohol solution of camphor. It should be stirred or ground quickly when added to prevent camphor from precipitating large particles due to solvent changes.

(4) Preparation of zinc sulfate solution: Weigh 3g of zinc sulfate, dissolve it in 25ml of water, and shake well.

III. Measurement of Sedimentation Volume Ratio and Redispersibility of Suspension

【Measurement of Sedimentation Volume Ratio】Put the calamine lotion of different prescriptions into 100ml measuring cylinders with stoppers, seal them tightly, and shake them for 1 minute, record the initial height H_0, stand them and timing, record the height H_u of the sedimentation at 5, 15, 30, 60, 90 and 120min, fill them in the Table 4-1, and calculate the settling volume ratio F. Note that the size and thickness of the measuring cylinders with stoppers are as consistent as possible.

【Re-dispersion experiment】Let the calamine lotion in different prescriptions stand for a period of time (one week or according to the actual situation) , turn the stopper cylinder upside down (one head and one tail is once) , and record the number of times required for re-dispersion of the sediment at the bottom of the test tube and fill the data in the Table 4-2. If the sediment at the bottom of the test tube is not dispersed all the time, record the result as "cake forming". The fewer times it takes to re-disperse the sediment at the bottom of the tube, the better redispersibility of the suspension.

 Results and Discussion

1. Results

(1) Drawing of settlement curve   According to the data in the Table 4-1, draw settlement curve with the sedimentation volume ratio F (H_u/H_0) for the ordinate and time (t) for the abscissa.

Table 4-1   Sedimentation volume ratio measurement results

Time/min	Calamine lotion									
	I		II		III		IV		V	
	H_u	F	H_u	F	H_u	F	H_u	F	H_u	F
5										
15										
30										
60										
90										
120										

(2) Re-dispersion experiment   The number of times required to re-disperse the sediment at the bottom of each test tube should be recorded in the Table 4-2.

Table 4-2   Re-dispersion times

Prescription	Calamine lotion				
	I	II	III	IV	V
Number of flips					

2. Discussions

(1) Analyze the effect of each stabilizer in calamine lotion.

(2) Compare calamine lotion and compound sulfur lotion. What is the difference of their preparation method?

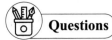 **Questions**

1. According to Stock's law and prescription, what are the main factors that affect the stability of suspensions?

2. What are the requirements for a good suspension?

3. Sulfur includes sublimated sulfur, refined sulfur, and precipitated sulfur. Why to choose precipitated sulfur in compound sulfur lotion?

PPT

实验五　注射液的制备及质量检查

实验目的

1. **掌握**　注射剂的制备工艺流程、操作要点及影响注射剂成品质量的因素。
2. **熟悉**　注射剂成品的质量检查内容及提高易氧化药物稳定性的基本方法。

实验原理

注射剂系指原料药与适宜的辅料制成的供注入体内的无菌制剂，可分为注射液（溶液型注射液、乳状液型注射液、混悬型注射液）、注射用无菌粉末与注射用浓溶液等。注射剂是目前临床尤其是急救诊疗应用中最广泛的剂型，其给药途径有皮内注射、皮下注射、肌内注射、静脉注射、脊椎腔注射、关节腔注射等。注射剂具有药效迅速、作用可靠；适用于不宜口服给药的药物；适用于不能口服给药的病人；可使药物发挥定位定向的局部作用等优点。但也存在注射时有疼痛感，患者依从性差；生产成本及质量要求高等缺点。

注射剂的处方由原料药、溶剂与附加剂组成。制备注射剂的原料药应符合注射用要求。注射剂的溶剂一般分为水性溶剂和非水性溶剂。注射用水是最常用的水性溶剂，蒸馏法是《中国药典》规定的制备注射用水的方法。对于不溶或难溶于水，或在水溶液中不稳定或有特殊用途的药物，可选用非水溶剂制备注射剂，常用的非水溶剂包括注射用油、乙醇、甘油、丙二醇、聚乙二醇等。

配制注射液时，可根据需要加入适宜的附加剂，常用的附加剂种类有抗氧剂、局麻剂、等渗调节剂、抑菌剂、pH调节剂、增溶剂、助溶剂、助悬剂、乳化剂等。一般多剂量注射剂、无菌操作法制备的注射剂可加适宜的抑菌剂，以防止注射剂制备过程中或使用过程中微生物的污染和生长繁殖。而静脉注射及脑池内、硬膜外、椎管内用的注射液均不得加抑菌剂，除另有规定外，一次注射量超过15ml的注射液也不得加抑菌剂。为防止注射剂由于主药的氧化产生的不稳定现象，可加入抗氧剂、惰性气体或金属络合剂。

注射剂常用容器有玻璃安瓿、玻璃瓶、塑料安瓿、塑料瓶（袋）、预装式注射器等。注射剂容器应符合有关注射用玻璃容器和塑料容器的国家标准的规定。

注射剂的制备工艺流程包括：原辅料的准备、配液、滤过、灌注、熔封、灭菌、质量检查、印字包装、成品等。用于制备注射剂的原辅料需使用注射用规格，配制前，应正确计算原料的用量。注射液的配制有浓配法和稀配法两种。配制所用的器具、原辅料尽可能无菌，配制时应在洁净的环境中进行，并尽可能缩短配制时间，以减少污染；对于不易过滤的药液可加0.1%~0.3%活性炭处理，亦可起到吸附热原、脱色等作用，但要注意其对药物的吸附作用。

药液配好后，要进行半成品的检查（pH、含量等），检查合格后才可进行滤过、灌封。滤过可除去不溶性的微粒，保持注射液的澄清，生产中通常采用二级过滤，先用常规滤器进行预滤，再用微孔滤膜精滤。灌封是注射剂制备的关键步骤，药液的灌注要求剂量准确，药液不沾瓶颈，对于接触空气不稳定的药液，可先往空容器中充入惰性气体，再灌装药液，药液填充后亦可再充一次惰性气体。安瓿封口的方法有顶封和拉封两种，工业生产中采用全自动灌封机。注射液在灌封后应尽快进行灭菌，一般注射剂从配制到灭菌不应超过 12 小时。对于稳定性良好的药物，目前普遍采用湿热灭菌法。灭菌后应立即进行检漏。

注射剂的质量要求主要包括：无菌、无热原，可见异物与不溶性微粒符合要求，pH、装量、渗透压和药物含量等应符合要求，在贮存期内应稳定有效。注射液的 pH 应接近体液，一般控制在 4~9 范围内；除另有规定外，静脉输液及椎管注射用注射液按各品种项下的规定，依照 2020 年版《中国药典》渗透压摩尔浓度测定法测定，应符合规定。除另有规定外，注射用无菌粉末的装量差异应符合规定。凡规定检查含量均匀度的品种，一般不再进行装量差异检查。此外，有些注射剂品种还需进行降压物质检查、异常毒性检查、刺激性和过敏性试验等。

实验器材

1. **仪器** 磁力搅拌器、pH 计、真空泵、微孔滤器、熔封机、灌装器、镊子、澄明度检查仪、紫外 - 可见分光光度计、烧杯、具塞三角瓶、玻璃漏斗、量筒、天平、电炉、称量纸、滤纸、脱脂棉、玻璃棒、牛角勺、安瓿、G₃ 垂熔漏斗、真空干燥箱等。

2. **材料** 维生素 C、碳酸氢钠、乙二胺四乙酸二钠（EDTA-2Na）、焦亚硫酸钠、注射用水、氮气、亚甲蓝等。

实验方法

（一）维生素 C 注射液的制备

【处方】

维生素 C	5.0g
碳酸氢钠	2.4g
乙二胺四乙酸二钠	0.005g
焦亚硫酸钠	0.2g
注射用水	加至 100ml

【制法】

（1）空安瓿的处理 空安瓿→灌水→处理→洗涤→干燥。

灌水、洗涤：将每支空安瓿灌满滤过的蒸馏水，以 100℃ 30 分钟热处理，甩水，再如上法灌水、甩水，反复两次。

干燥：将洗好的安瓿置真空干燥箱内 120℃温度下干燥 2 小时，备用。

（2）注射液的配制 按处方取配制量 80% 的注射用水，通入 N₂ 饱和；称取并加入维生素 C 溶解后，分次缓缓地加入碳酸氢钠，搅拌待完全溶解后，调节药液 pH 5.8~6.2；加入乙二胺四乙酸二钠、焦亚硫酸钠溶解，添加 N₂ 饱和的注射用水至足量，用 G₃ 垂熔漏斗预滤，再用 0.22μm 的微孔滤膜精滤；检查滤液澄明度合格后，即可灌封。

（3）灌注与熔封 将过滤合格的药液，立即灌装于 2ml 安瓿中，要求装量准确，药液不得沾安瓿颈壁，并通 N₂ 于安瓿上部空间，随灌随封。熔封后的安瓿顶部应圆滑、无尖头、鼓泡或凹陷现象。

（4）灭菌与检漏 将灌封好的安瓿用 100℃流通蒸汽灭菌 15 分钟；灭菌完毕立即将安瓿放入 1% 亚甲蓝水溶液中，剔除变色安瓿，将合格安瓿洗净、擦干，供质量检查用。

【性状】本品为无色至微黄色的澄明液体。

【注意事项】

（1）维生素 C 的性质极不稳定，分子中在羰基毗邻的位置上有两个烯醇基，在水溶液中极易被氧化，其内酯环结构容易水解。维生素 C 注射液发生变黄的原因，可能是自身氧化水解生成的或由原料中带入的呋喃甲醛在空气中继续氧化聚合呈黄色。因此生产中采取通入 N_2、调节药液 pH、添加抗氧剂及金属络合剂等措施。此外，在制备过程中应避免与金属用具接触。

（2）维生素 C 显强酸性，加入碳酸氢钠可使部分维生素 C 中和成钠盐，提高本品的稳定性，又可避免酸性太强，在注射时产生疼痛；将碳酸氢钠加入维生素 C 溶液中时速度要慢，以防止产生大量气泡使溶液溢出，同时要不断搅拌，以防局部碱性过强，造成维生素 C 的破坏。

（3）熔封时需调节火焰，要求火焰细而有力，燃烧完全，双焰灯两火焰应有一定的夹角，火焰交点处温度最高，可将安瓿颈部置于火焰温度最高处熔封，并掌握好安瓿在火焰中停留的时间。

（二）质量检查

【颜色】 照 2020 年版《中国药典》溶液颜色检查法进行检查。取本品，加水稀释成每 1ml 中含维生素 C 50mg 的溶液，照紫外 - 可见分光光度法，在 420nm 波长处测定，吸收度不得低于 0.06。

【装量】 照 2020 年版《中国药典》装量检查法进行检查。取供试品 5 支（每支 2ml），开启时注意避免损失，将内容物分别用相应体积的干燥注射器及注射针头抽尽，再缓慢连续地注入经标化的量入式量筒内，在室温下检视。每支的装量均不得少于其标示量。

【pH】 应为 5.0~7.0。

【可见异物检查】 照 2020 年版《中国药典》可见异物检查法进行检查。除特殊规定外，注射剂不得含有任何肉眼可见的不溶性微粒异物。采用人工灯检法，在暗室中进行。灯检法的装置为带有遮光板的日光灯光源（光照度可在 1000~4000lx 范围内调节）；不反光的黑色背景；不反光的白色背景和底部（供检查有色异物）；反光的白色背景（指遮光板内侧）。取供试品 20 支，除去容器标签，擦净容器外壁，必要时将药液转移至洁净透明的适宜容器内，将供试品置遮光板边缘处，在明视距离（指供试品至人眼的清晰观测距离，通常为 25cm），手持容器颈部，轻轻旋转和翻转容器（但应避免产生气泡），使药液中可能存在的可见异物悬浮，分别在黑色和白色背景下目视检查，重复观察，总检查时限为 20 秒。供试品装量每支在 10ml 及 10ml 以下的，每次检查可手持 2 支。供试品溶液中有大量气泡产生影响观察时，需静置足够时间至气泡消失后检查。

💬 **实验结果与讨论**

1. **维生素 C 注射液质量检查** 　将维生素 C 注射液颜色、装量、pH、可见异物检查结果填于表 5-1。

表 5-1　维生素 C 注射液质量检查结果

检查项目	颜色	装量	pH	可见异物
检查结果				
结果判断				

2. **讨论** 　维生素 C 注射液可能产生的质量问题是什么？应如何控制工艺过程？

思考题

1. 影响注射剂澄明度的因素有哪些？
2. 试述注射剂污染热原的途径及除去注射剂中热原的方法。
3. 试述注射剂各类附加剂的作用及常用品种。
4. 制备注射用水的常用方法和设备有哪些？

（颜　红）

Lab. 5　Preparation and Quality Inspection of Injections

 Experimental Objectives

1. To master the preparation process, operation points of injection and the factors affecting the quality of final injection products.

2. To be familiar with the quality control of the final injection and the basic methods to improve the stability of easily oxidizable drugs.

 Experimental Principles

Injections are sterile products using drug substances with suitable excipients which are intended to be injected into the body, and can be classified into liquids for injection (solutions, emulsions and suspensions), sterilized powders for injection and concentrated solutions for injection, etc.. Injections are currently the most widely used form in clinical applications, especially for emergency diagnosis and treatment, which can be applied to intracutaneous, subcutaneous, intramuscular, intravenous, spinal cavity and intra-articular injecting administrations, etc. With the advantages of rapid therapeutic efficacy and reliable effects, the injections are usually in the drugs that are not suitable for oral administration and can be used for patients who can't be administered orally, which can make the drug play the role of localization and orientation. However, there are also disadvantages such as pain during injection, poor patient's compliance, high production costs and quality requirements, etc.

The formula of injections consists of drug substances, solvents and excipients, and the drug substances prepared for injections should comply with the requirements for injection. The solvents for injections are generally divided into aqueous solvents and non-aqueous solvents. Water for injection is the most commonly-used aqueous solvents and distillation is the method for preparation of water for injection as prescribed in the *Chinese Pharmacopoeia*. For drugs that are insoluble or hardly soluble in water, or are unstable in aqueous solutions or have special uses, non-aqueous solvents can be used to prepare injections. Commonly-used non-aqueous solvents include oil for injection, ethanol, glycerol, propanediol and polyethylene glycol, etc.

Suitable additives may be added according to the need. The common additives include antioxidants, local anesthetics, isotonic regulators, antimicrobial preservatives, pH regulators, solubilizers, hydrotropic agents, suspending agents, emulsifying agents, etc. Generally multi-dose injections and injections prepared by aseptic manipulation may contain an appropriate concentration of antimicrobial preservatives to prevent the contamination, growth and reproduction of micro-organisms during the preparation or use of the injections. It is not allowed to use antimicrobial preservatives for injections to be administered by intravenous injection, intracisternal injection, extradural injection or vertebral canula injection. Unless otherwise specified, antimicrobial preservatives can't be added to the injections with a single dose

36

of more than 15ml. To prevent the instability of the injections due to the oxidation of the main drug, antioxidants, inert gas or metal complexing agents can be added.

Commonly-used containers for injections include glass ampoules, glass bottles, plastic ampoules, plastic bottles (bags) and prefilled syringes, etc. Containers should comply with the related requirements of the National Standards for glass and plastic containers for injections.

The preparation procedure of the injections includes: Preparation of raw materials, blending, filtration, filling, sealing by fusion, sterilization, quality inspection, printing and packaging, finished products and so on. The raw materials for preparation of injections should meet the specifications for injection, and their amounts should be calculated correctly before preparation. Concentrated preparation and diluted preparation are the two methods for preparation of injections. The Equipments and raw materials used in the preparation are as sterile as possible; the preparation should be performed in a clean environment, and the preparation time should be reduced as far as possible to avoid contamination; the drug solution that is not easy to filter can be treated with 0.1% to 0.3% activated carbon, which can also play the role of adsorption of pyrogens and decoloration, but attention should be paid to its adsorption effects on drugs.

After preparing the drug solution, the semi-finished product should be inspected (pH value, content, etc.), and then filtered, filled and sealed. Filtration can remove the insoluble particles and keep the injections clear. Two-stage filtration is usually adopted in producing. Pre-filtration with conventional filter first, then refined filtration with millipore filter. Filling and sealing are the key steps in the preparation of injections. The dosage should be accurate and the drug solution does not stick to the bottle neck during filling. For the drug solution that is unstable in contact with air, the empty container can be filled with insert gas firstly, followed by the drug solution and then the inert gas again. There are two sealing methods of ampoule: top sealing and pull, sealing. Full-automatic filling and sealing machines are used in the industrial production. The injections should be sterilized as soon as possible after filling and sealing. Generally, it should not exceed 12 hours from preparation to sterilization. Moist heat sterilization is currently widely used for drugs with good stability. Leak detection should be performed immediately after sterilization.

The quality requirements of injections mainly include: sterile, pyrogen-free; visible particles and insoluble particles should meet the requirements; pH value, filling amount, osmotic pressure and drug content should meet the requirements, and the injections should be stable and effective during storage. The pH value of the injections should be close to the body fluid, and generally controlled within the range of 4~9. Unless otherwise specified, the injections for intravenous infusion or vertebral canula injections should comply with the requirements of the Determination of Osmolarity in the *Chinese Pharmacopoeia* (2020). Unless otherwise specified, the difference in the filling amount of sterile powders for injection should meet the requirements. For varieties that require the uniformity of content, the inspection of the difference in filling amount is generally not performed. In addition, some varieties of the injections also need to be tested for hypotensive substance, abnormal toxicity, irritation and hypersensitivity.

Equipments and Materials

1. Equipments Magnetic stirrer, pH meter, vacuum pump, millipore filter, fusion sealer, filler, tweezers, clarity tester, UV-visible spectrophotometer, beaker, conical flask with stopper, glass funnel, graduated cylinder, balance, electric furnace, weighing paper, filter paper, absorbent cotton, glass rod, horn spoon, ampoule, G₃ sintered filter funnel, vacuum drying oven, etc.

2. Materials Vitamin C, sodium bicarbonate, ethylene diamine tetraacetic acid (EDTA–2Na), sodium metabisulfite, water for injection, nitrogen, methylene blue, etc.

Experimental Methods

I. Preparation of Vitamin C Injections

【Formula】

Vitamin C	5.0g
Sodium bicarbonate	2.4g
EDTA–2Na	0.005g
Sodium metabisulfite	0.2g
Water for injection	Add to 100ml

【Procedure】

(1) Treatment of empty ampoule: Empty ampoule → water filling → treatment → washing → drying.

Water filling and washing: After being filled with filtered distilled water, each empty ampoule receives heat treatment at 100℃ for 30 minutes, followed by shaking water off, and repeats twice as above.

Drying: The washed ampoules are placed in a vacuum drying oven at 120℃ for 2 hours and set aside.

(2) Preparation of injections: Take 80% of water for injection according to the formula, and be saturated with N_2; weight and add Vitamin C to dissolve, slowly add sodium bicarbonate for several times, stir until well dissolved, adjust the pH value of the solution to 5.8~6.2; add EDTA–2Na and sodium metabisulfite to dissolve, and N_2 saturated water for injection to a sufficient amount; take pre-filtration with a G₃ sintered filter funnel, and then refined filtration with a 0.22μm millipore membrane; after checking the clarity of filtrate qualified, filling and sealing can be conducted.

(3) Filling and fusion sealing: Fill the qualified filtered drug solution into 2ml ampoules immediately; the filling amount should be accurate, and the drug solution shall not touch the neck wall of the ampoule. Fill the upper space of ampoule with N_2; seal immediately after filling; the top of sealed ampoule by fusion should be smooth, free from sharp tips, blisters or dents.

(4) Sterilization and leak test: Sterilize the sealed ampoule with 100℃ flowing steam for 15 min; after sterilization, immediately place the ampoule in the 1% methylene blue solution; remove the discolored ampoules, wash and dry the qualified ampoules for quality inspection.

【Description】Colorless to light yellow clear liquid.

【Notes】

(1) Vitamin C is extremely unstable in nature. There are two enoyl groups adjacent to the carbonyl group in the molecule, which is easily oxidized in the aqueous solution, and its lactone ring structure is easily hydrolyzed. The yellowing of Vitamin C injections may be due to furfural formed by auto-oxidative hydrolysis or carried by the raw materials, which continues to oxidize and polymerize to yellow in the air. Therefore, measures such as introducing N_2, regulating pH value of the drug solution, adding antioxidants and metal complexing agents are adopted in the production. In addition, avoid contact with metal appliances during preparation.

(2) Vitamin C is strongly acidic. Sodium bicarbonate can be added to neutralize part of Vitamin C into sodium salts, improve the stability of the product, and avoid being too acidic, which can cause pain during injection; slowly add sodium bicarbonate to Vitamin C solution to prevent formation of a large number of bubbles causing the solution to overflow, meanwhile keep stirring to prevent local alkalinity from being too high and causing destruction of Vitamin C.

(3) Regulate the flame when sealing by fusion. The flame should be fine and powerful, and burn completely. The two flames of a double flame lamp should have a certain angle. The temperature at the flame intersection is the highest. The neck of the ampoule can be placed at the highest temperature of the flame for sealing by fusion, and the time of ampoules staying in the flame should be controlled.

II. Quality Inspection

【Color】Check color of the solution according to the test method listed in the *Chinese Pharmacopoeia* (2020). Take the product for diluting with water into a solution containing 50mg of Vitamin C per 1ml, and measure it at wavelength of 420nm by UV-spectrophotometry. The absorbance shall not be less than 0.06.

【Filling】Comply with the relevant provisions under the Checking Minimum Loading Capacity in the *Chinese Pharmacopoeia* (2020). Take 5 containers (each 2ml), open the container cautiously to avoid any loss of the contents. Take up individually the content of each container into a dry syringe, then discharge the content of the syringe into a caliberated cylinder slowly and continuously, and measure the volume at room temperature. The content in each container is not less than the labeled quantity of the injection.

【pH value】The pH value should be 5.0~7.0.

【Test for visible particles】Comply with the requirements of the Test for Visible Particles in the *Chinese Pharmacopoeia* (2020). Unless otherwise specified, the injection shall not contain any insoluble particulate foreign matter visible to the naked eye. Lamp test is the commonly used method which carried out in a darkroom. The apparatus for lamp test includes a light source of daylight lamp with panel for obstructing from light (the intensity of illumination is adjustable between 1000~4000 lx), a non-glare black background, a non-glare white background and the bottom (supply with test for colored particles), a glare white background (inboard of light baffle) as well. Take 20 containers, remove any adherent labels from the containers, clean the outer surface. If necessary, transfer the solution being examined into another clean and diaphanous appropriative glass container. Hold the bootle-neck of the container at the edge of light baffle, gently swirl and invert the container in order to force the visible particles in the solution being examined floating (ensuring that air bubbles are not introduced), meanwhile observe any insoluble substances in the container and keep appropriate distance from inspector's eyes to the container (It's usually 25cm to inspect clearly) with visual method respectively in front of black background and white background. Repeat several times within 20 seconds. Hold 2 ampoules (vials) for each observation if the volume of solution being examined is not more than 10ml per ampoule (vial). If a large number of air bubbles are introduced, the solution should allow to stand for sufficient time before examination until bubbles disappear.

Results and Discussions

1. Results　Record the inspection results of color, filling amount, pH value and visible particles for Vitamin C injections in the Table 5–1.

Table 5—1   Results of quality inspection for vitamin C injections

Inspection items	Color	Filling amount	pH value	Visible particles
Inspection results				
Results judgement				

2. Discussions   What are the possible quality problems with Vitamin C injections?   How should the process be controlled?

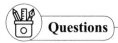 **Questions**

1. What are the factors affecting the clarity of the injections?

2. Describe the ways to contaminate injections by pyrogens and the methods to remove pyrogens from injections.

3. Describe the functions of various additives and common types of injections.

4. What are the common methods and Equipments for preparing water for injection?

实验六 滴眼剂的制备

PPT

实验目的

1. **掌握** 滴眼剂的制备工艺流程及质量检查方法。
2. **熟悉** 滴眼剂常用附加剂种类及等渗调节的方法。

实验原理

　　滴眼剂是指原料药与适宜辅料制成的无菌水性或油性澄明溶液、混悬液或乳状液，供滴入眼部的液体制剂。滴眼剂用于眼黏膜，每次用量1~2滴，起杀菌、消炎、扩瞳、局部麻醉等作用。滴眼剂虽属外用制剂，由于给药部位比较特殊，因此，其制备方法和质量标准的要求相对严格，近似于注射剂。

　　一般滴眼剂为多剂量包装，反复使用过程中与环境及病眼接触，易造成污染，需加抑菌剂。一般滴眼剂要求无致病菌，尤其不得检出铜绿假单胞菌和金黄色葡萄球菌。用于眼外伤及手术的滴眼剂不宜加抑菌剂，应严格灭菌，采用单剂量包装。

　　药物耐热的滴眼剂制备流程为：

$$\left.\begin{array}{l} 原料药及辅料预处理 \rightarrow 配液 \rightarrow 过滤 \rightarrow 灭菌 \\ 瓶、塞 \rightarrow 洗涤 \rightarrow 灭菌 \end{array}\right\} 无菌分装 \rightarrow 质检 \rightarrow 印字 \rightarrow 包装$$

实验器材

1. **仪器** 电子天平、温度计，烧杯、G_3垂熔玻璃漏斗、输液瓶、滴眼剂瓶（10ml）、灌注器、灭菌器、澄明度检测仪、无菌操作柜等。

2. **材料** 氯霉素、硼砂、硼酸、羟苯乙酯、羟丙甲纤维素（MW4500）、氯化钠、苯扎氯铵溶液、注射用水等。

实验方法

（一）氯霉素滴眼液的制备

【处方】

氯霉素	0.25g
硼砂	0.3g
硼酸	1.9g
羟苯乙酯	0.03g
注射用水	加至 100ml

【制法】

（1）容器的处理　塑料滴眼剂瓶先用 75% 乙醇吸入消毒，再用注射用水洗至无醇味，沥干备用。

（2）配液　称取硼酸、硼砂溶于约 90ml 的热注射用水中（90℃左右），然后加入氯霉素与羟苯乙酯，搅拌溶解，加注射用水至 100ml，调 pH 在 6~8，用 G₃ 垂熔玻璃漏斗过滤至澄明，滤液灌封于干净的输液瓶中，煮沸灭菌 30 分钟。

（3）无菌分装　在无菌操作柜内将灭菌的氯霉素溶液分装于滴眼瓶中，密封，加塞，印字包装即得。

【性状】本品应为无色或近无色的澄明液体。

【用途】用于急、慢性结膜炎，以及沙眼、角膜炎和眼睑缘炎。

【注意事项】

（1）处方中加硼砂、硼酸做缓冲剂，调节 pH 和渗透压，同时还可增加氯霉素的溶解度。本品在 pH 约为 6 时最稳定。

（2）氯霉素对热较稳定，故配液时可加热以加速溶解。

（3）本品中羟苯乙酯（0.02%）为抑菌剂。

（二）人工泪液的制备

【处方】

羟丙甲纤维素（MW4500）	0.3g
氯化钠	0.37g
苯扎氯铵溶液	0.02ml
硼砂	0.19g
硼酸	0.19g
氯化钾	0.45g
注射用水	加至 100ml

【制法】

（1）容器的处理　塑料滴眼瓶先用 75% 乙醇吸入消毒，再用注射用水洗至无醇味，沥干备用。

（2）配液　称取羟丙甲基纤维素溶于适量注射用水中，依次加入硼砂、硼酸、氯化钠、氯化钾、苯扎氯铵溶液，添加注射用水至全量，搅拌均匀，调 pH 在 6~8 范围内，用 G₃ 垂熔玻璃漏斗过滤至澄明，滤液灌封于干净的输液瓶中，煮沸法灭菌 30 分钟。

（3）无菌分装　在无菌操作柜内将灭菌的人工泪液分装于滴眼剂瓶中，密封，加塞，印字包装即得。

【性状】本品为无色澄明液体。

【用途】滋润眼睛，消除眼部不适，治疗眼干燥症。

【注意事项】

（1）羟丙甲纤维素为增稠剂，其 2% 溶液在 20℃时的黏度为 3750~5250mPa·s。

（2）处方中的苯扎氯铵溶液系苯扎氯铵的 50% 水溶液。

实验结果与讨论

1. 结果　将氯霉素滴眼液、人工泪液的性状检查结果填入表 6-1 中。

表 6-1　滴眼液的性状检查结果

制剂	颜色	嗅味	澄明度	pH
氯霉素滴眼液				
人工泪液				

2. 讨论

（1）处方中硼酸、硼砂、羟苯乙酯各起什么作用？

（2）分析产品质量情况，讨论影响产品质量的关键实验步骤。

思考题

1. 结合本实验的处方，讨论滴眼剂处方设计应考虑的问题。

2. 滴眼剂中选择抑菌剂应考虑哪些问题？

3. 调节 pH 和渗透压时应注意哪些方面？

（蔡邦荣）

Lab. 6 Preparation of Eye Drops

Experimental Objectives

1. To master the preparation process of eye drops and their quality inspection methods.
2. To be familiar with the types of common additives and the methods of isotonic adjustment of eye drops.

Experimental Principles

Eye drops are sterile liquid preparations dripped into the eye made of raw materials and suitable excipients, including sterile aqueous or oily transparent solution, suspensions, or emulsions. Eye drops are dripped into the mucous membrane of the eye, with the dosage of 1~2 drops each time, which have the functions of disinfection, anti-inflammation, widening the pupil, and topical anesthesia, etc.. As the eye is an extremely delicate organ, preparation methods and quality standards of eye drops are relatively strict, which are close to those of injection preparations although they belong to external preparation.

Eye drops are generally packaged in a multi-dose system. They are easily contaminated by the bacteria exposed to air or contacting with eyes once opened, preservative is thereby added in the eye drops to ensure eye drops free from pathogenic bacteria, especially pseudomonas aeruginosa and staphylococcus aureus. Eye drops for ocular injury and surgery are not suitable to adding preservative, and should be strictly sterilized and packed in single dose.

The preparation procedure of eye drops containing heat-resistant drugs is as following:

Pretreatment of drugs and additives→preparation of solution→filtration→terilization }
Bottle and seal→washing→sterilization }
→aseptic packaging→quality inspection→embossing→packaging

Equipments and Materials

1. Equipments Balance, thermometer, beakers, glass funnel with G_3, dropping bottle, 10ml plastic empty dropper bottles with tip cap, syringe, sterilizer, transparency tester, biosafety cabinet, etc.

2. Materials Chloramphenicol (CHL), borax, boric acid, nipagin, sodium chloride, potassium chloride, hydroxypropyl methylcellulose (HPMC, MW 4500), benzalkonium chloride solution, and water for injection, etc.

Experimental Methods

I. Preparation of Chloramphenicol Eye Drops

【Formula】

Chloramphenicol 0.25g

Borax	0.3g
Boric acid	1.9g
Nipagin	0.03g
Water for injection	Add to 100ml

【Procedure】

(1) Container handling, suck 75% ethanol into the plastic empty dropper bottles for sterilization, followed by washing with the water for injection till no alcohol taste and draining off.

(2) Solution preparation, borax and boric acid are dissolved into 90ml pre-heated sterilized water (around 90℃), followed by addition of CHL and nipagin with frequent agitation till completely dissolved, fill the water for injection up to 100ml and adjust pH value in the range of 6 to 8. The resulting solution is filtrated by the glass funnel with G_3 to give transparent solution, the filtrate is transferred into the pre-treated dropping bottles. After that, the bottles are sealed and placed into a boiling water bather over 30min for sterilization.

(3) The obtained solution of CHL is packaged into eye dropper bottle in the biosafety cabinet, followed by heat-sealing, capping, sealing, embossing and packaging to get the final product.

【Description】Transparent colorless or close colorless liquid.

【Application】Acute or chronic conjunctivitis, trachoma, keratitis and peripetalitis.

【Notes】

(1) Since CHL has superior stability of pH 6 in aqueous solution, borax-boric acid act as buffer system to adjust pH and osmotic pressure. It can also increase the solubility of CHL.

(2) Thanks to better thermal stability of CHL, it can be heated in a water bather to accelerate its dissolution.

(3) Nipagin (0.02%, *w/v*) is a preservative in the formulation.

II. Preparation of Artificial Tears

【Prescription】

HPMC (MW 4500)	0.3g
NaCl	0.37g
Benzalkonium chloride solution	0.02ml
KCl	0.45g
Borax	0.19g
Boric acid	0.19g
Water for injection	Add to 100ml

【Procedure】

(1) Container handling, suck 75% ethanol into the plastic empty dropper bottles for sterilization, wash by the water for injection till no alcohol taste and draining off.

(2) Solution preparation, dissolve HPMC in a moderate amount of water for injection, followed by adding boric acid, borax, NaCl, KCl and benzalkonium chloride solution, fill the water for injection up to 100ml, mix well the resulting solution and adjust its pH ranging from 6 to 8. The obtained solution is filtrated by the glass funnel with G_3 sand core filter to give transparent solution, the filtrate is completely transferred into the pre-treated dropping bottle. After that, bottles are sealed and placed into a boiling water bather over 30min for sterilization.

(3) The sterilized artificial tears are packed into eye dropper bottle in the biosafety cabinet, followed by heat-sealing, capping, sealing, embossing and packaging to give the final product.

【Description】Transparent colorless liquid.

【Application】Moisten the eyes, relieve eye discomfort caused by dry eye, and treat dry eye syndrome.

【Notes】

(1) HPMC acts as a thickening agent and the 2% (*w/v*) solution of which has a viscosity range of 3750~5250mPa · s at 20℃.

(2) Benzalkonium chloride solution refers to benzalkonium chloride 50% (*w/v*) in aqueous solution.

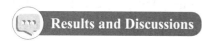 **Results and Discussions**

1. Results Record the quality in terms of color, odor, solution appearance and pH for these eye drops in the Table 6–1.

Table 6–1　Results of quality inspection for eye drops

Preparations	Color	Odor	Solution appearance (clarity)	pH
Chloramphenicol eye drops				
Artifical tears				

2. Discussions

(1) What are the roles that boric acid, borax and nipagin play in the formula?

(2) Analyze the results and discuss key factors that affect the formulation quality.

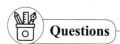 **Questions**

1. Based on above experiments, what issues need to pay attention in prescription design for eye drops?

2. What should be considered when choosing preservatives for eye drops?

3. What should be noticed when adjusting pH and osmoticpressure?

PPT

实验七　散剂的制备

实验目的

1. **掌握**　散剂的制备方法及等量递增混合方法。
2. **熟悉**　散剂的常规质量检查方法。

实验原理

散剂是指原料药或与适宜的辅料经粉碎、均匀混合制成的干燥粉末状制剂，供口服或局部用药。按药物性质可分为一般散剂、含毒性成分散剂、含液体成分散剂、含低共熔成分散剂。散剂应干燥、疏松、混合均匀、色泽一致，且装量差异、装量、干燥失重或水分、微生物限度检查应符合规定。一般内服散剂，应通过 5~6 号筛；用于消化道溃疡病的散剂、儿科和外用散剂应通过 7 号筛；眼用散剂则应通过 9 号筛。

散剂的制备工艺流程：粉碎→过筛→混合→分剂量→质量检查→包装。

散剂制法简便，其中混合操作是关键环节。目前常用的混合方法有搅拌混合、研磨混合、过筛混合等。混合均匀度是散剂质量的重要指标，含有少量毒性药品及贵重药品的散剂，为保证混合均匀，应采用等量递加法（配研法）混合；含有少量挥发油及共熔成分的散剂，可先用处方中其他固体成分吸收，再与其他成分混合。散剂一般采取密封包装与密闭贮藏，避免贮藏过程中吸潮、变质。

实验器材

1. **仪器**　研钵、天平、药筛等。
2. **材料**　麝香草酚、薄荷脑、薄荷油、樟脑、水杨酸、升华硫、硼酸、氧化锌、淀粉、滑石粉、硫酸阿托品、胭脂红、乳糖等。

实验方法

（一）痱子粉的制备

【处方】

麝香草酚	0.6g
薄荷脑	0.6g
薄荷油	0.6ml
樟脑	0.6g
水杨酸	1.4g
升华硫	4.0g

硼酸	8.5g
氧化锌	6.0g
淀粉	10.0g
滑石粉	加至 100.0g

【制备】

（1）取麝香草酚、薄荷脑、樟脑研磨共熔，与薄荷油混匀。

（2）另将水杨酸、硼酸、氧化锌、升华硫及淀粉分别研细，混匀；用混合细粉吸收上述混合液，充分研匀。

（3）按等量递增法加入滑石粉研匀，使成 100g，过 7 号筛，即得。

【性状】本品为白色粉末；气香。

【用途】散风除湿，清凉止痒。用于汗疹，痱毒。

【注意事项】制备时先将麝香草酚、薄荷脑、樟脑制成低共熔物。

（二）硫酸阿托品散（倍散）的制备

【处方】

硫酸阿托品	0.1g
1% 胭脂红乳糖	0.1g
乳糖	9.8g

【制备】先取少量乳糖饱和研钵表面能；将硫酸阿托品与胭脂红乳糖研磨混匀，再以等量递增法分次加入乳糖研匀，即得。

【性状】本品为浅红色的粉末。

【作用与用途】抗胆碱药，常用于胃肠痉挛、疼痛等。

【注意事项】

（1）先用乳糖饱和研钵，以防吸附药物、影响剂量。

（2）1% 胭脂红乳糖的配制：取胭脂红 1g 置研钵内，加入 90% 乙醇 10~20ml 研磨使其溶解，加入少量乳糖吸收，再按照等量递增法分次加入剩余乳糖（总量 99g）研匀直至色泽均匀；50~60℃下干燥，过 6 号筛，即得。

（3）利用胭脂红着色，不仅方便观察混合程度，也利于辨别不同稀释程度的倍散。

（4）本品中硫酸阿托品有毒、量少，宜采用重量法分剂量。

💬 实验结果与讨论

1. **结果**　将痱子粉、硫酸阿托品散的性状检查结果分别填入表 7-1。

表 7-1　散剂质量检查结果

药品	性状	均匀度	气味
痱子粉			
硫酸阿托品散			

2. **讨论**　分析产品质量情况，讨论影响产品质量的主要实验步骤。

思考题

1. 等量递增法的原则是什么?

2. 何谓低共熔? 常见的低共熔组分有哪些?

3. 制备倍散的目的是什么? 处方中一般应包含哪些组分? 在混合操作中应注意哪些问题?

（王文苹）

Lab. 7 Preparation of Powders

 Experimental Objectives

1. To master methods for preparation of powders and the equivalent incremental method.
2. To be familiar with methods commonly used for quality control of powders.

 Experimental Principles

Powders are preparations in dry powder state, prepared by comminuting and homogeneously mixing active ingredients with suitable excipients for oral or topical medication. In terms of drug properties, powders can be basically categorized into common powders, powders with toxic drugs, powders with liquid drugs, and powders with eutectic components. The powders must be homogeneously mixed and dry, with uniform color and loose appearance, also meet the requirements on filling variation, water content and microbial limit test. Common powders for internal administration have to pass through No.5 or No.6 sieve. And No.7 sieve for powders of ulcer treatment of digestive tract and pediatric or topical application, No.9 sieve for powders of ophthalmic application.

The production process of powders is shown as follows: Comminution→sieving→mixing→dosing→ quality control→packaging.

The preparation method of powders is simple and mixing is the critical process. Commonly used mixing methods include stirring, grinding and sieving. Mixing uniformity is one of the key index of powder quality. The equivalent incremental method (also called geometric dilution method) is suitable for preparation of powders with a low dose of toxic or costly drugs. The volatile oil or eutectic components in the formulation should be absorbed using some solid ingredients before mixing with other ingredients. Usually, the powders should be preserved in sealed package and airtight storage to avoid moisture absorption or deterioration.

 Equipments and Materials

1. Equipments   Mortar, balance, sieve, etc.

2. Materials   Thymol, menthol, mint oil, camphor, salicylic acid, sublimed sulfur, boric acid, zinc oxide, starch, talc, atropine sulfate, carmine, lactose, etc.

 Experimental Methods

Ⅰ. Preparation of Anti-rash Powders

【 Formula 】

Thymol   0.6g

Menthol	0.6g
Mint oil	0.6ml
Camphor	0.6g
Salicylic acid	1.4g
Sublimed sulfur	4.0g
Boric acid	8.5g
Zinc oxide	6.0g
Starch	10.0g
Talc	Add to 100.0g

【Procedure】

(1) Grind together thymol, menthol and camphor in the mortar until completely melt, and homogeneously mix with mint oil.

(2) Grind salicylic acid, boric acid, zinc oxide, sublimed sulfur and starch individually to be fine powders, and mix them together. The powder is further blended with the obtained mixture solution to form homogeneous powders.

(3) Add talc using the equivalent incremental method and finally pass through a No.7 sieve.

【Description】 A white powder with cool smell.

【Application】 Dispel wind and dampness, cool skin and relieve itching. Commonly used for sweet rash and heat poison.

【Note】 Firstly mix thymol, menthol and camphor to form eutectic liquid during the process.

II. Preparation of Atropine Sulfate Powders (exponentially diluted powders)

【Formula】

Atropine sulfate	0.1g
1% Carmine-dyed lactose	0.1g
Lactose	9.8g

【Procedure】 Firstly, saturate the inner surface of a mortar by grinding with a small amount of lactose. Then mix together atropine sulfate and carmine-dyed lactose in the mortar. Add lactose using geometric dilution method to make the final product homogeneous.

【Description】 A light pink powder.

【Application】 Anticholinergic agent, commonly used for gastrointestinal spasm and pain.

【Note】

(1) Saturation of the mortar with lactose before mixing is aimed to prevent drug adsorption and dose inaccuracy.

(2) Preparation of 1% carmine-dyed lactose: Dissolve 1g carmine into 10~20ml of 90% ethanol in the mortar. Absorb the solution by a small amount of lactose, and then add the rest of lactose (99g in total) using the geometric dilution method. Grind the mixture to obtain a uniform appearance. Dry the powder at 50~60℃ and pass through a No.6 sieve.

(3) Dyeing with carmine is beneficial to observe the uniformity of mixture and differentiate powders with different dilution degrees.

(4) Atropine sulfate is toxic and at a low dose. Therefore, the final product is recommended to be divided by weight.

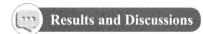

Results and Discussions

1. Results Record the inspection results in the Table 7–1.

Table 7–1 Results of quality inspection for powders

Preparations	Property description	Uniformity	Odor
Anti-rash powder			
Atropine sulfate powder			

2. Discussions Analyze the results and discuss the key factors influencing the products quality.

 Questions

1. What is the principle of equivalent incremental method?

2. What is eutectic phenomenon and list commonly-used eutectic components?

3. What is the aim for preparation of exponentially diluted powders, what kinds of components are suitable for this formulation and what issues should be paid attention to in mixing process?

实验八　片剂的制备及质量检查

PPT

实验目的

1. **掌握** 湿法制粒压片的制备方法。
2. **熟悉** 片剂重量差异、硬度、脆碎度、崩解时限、溶出度等质量检查方法。
3. **了解** 压片机的结构及工作原理。

实验原理

片剂系指药物与辅料制成的圆形或异形的片状固体制剂。口服用片剂有普通压制片、糖衣片、薄膜衣片、肠溶片、咀嚼片、分散片、泡腾片、口腔速崩片或口腔速溶片、缓释片、控释片及多层片等，口腔用片剂有舌下片、含片、口腔贴片，外用片剂有溶液片、阴道片与阴道泡腾片。片剂是现代医疗中应用最广泛的剂型之一。

片剂的辅料按作用可分为稀释剂、吸收剂、润湿剂、黏合剂、崩解剂、抗黏剂、助流剂、润滑剂等。常用的稀释剂有淀粉、糖粉、糊精、乳糖、可压性淀粉、微晶纤维素等；吸收剂有硫酸钙、磷酸氢钙等；润湿剂有水、乙醇；黏合剂有淀粉浆、纤维素衍生物、聚维酮、聚乙二醇、明胶、糖浆等；崩解剂有干淀粉、羧甲淀粉钠、低取代羟丙基纤维素、交联羧甲基纤维素钠、交联聚维酮、泡腾崩解剂等；润滑剂有硬脂酸镁、微粉硅胶、滑石粉、氢化植物油、月桂醇硫酸钠（镁）等；此外，片剂的辅料还有着色剂、矫味剂等。

片剂的制备方法可分为湿法制粒压片、干法制粒压片和粉末直接压片三种，除对湿、热不稳定的药物外，多数药物采用湿法制粒压片，其工艺流程为：

粉碎→过筛→混合→制软材→制粒→干燥→整粒→总混→压片→（包衣）→包装

制粒的方法有挤出制粒、高速搅拌制粒、流化床制粒、喷雾制粒等方法，实验室通常采用挤出制粒的方式。

片剂制备过程中的注意事项：①原料药与辅料应混合均匀。②制粒与压片是片剂制备的关键工序，颗粒形状、大小、含水量及压缩特性等均会影响压片过程的进行和片剂质量；片剂应具有适宜的硬度，以保证片剂外观形状及崩解要求。③具有挥发性或遇热易分解的药物，在制片过程中应避免受热损失。④压片时压力应适度，保证片剂有一定的硬度。⑤具有不适的臭味、刺激性、易潮解或遇光易变质的药物，制成片剂后，可包糖衣或薄膜衣；遇胃液易破坏或需要在肠内释放的药物，可制成肠溶衣片。

制成的片剂应进行质量检查，包括性状、重量差异、硬度、脆碎度、崩解时限、含量均匀度、溶出度、释放度等。《中国药典》要求，凡规定检查含量均匀度的片剂，一般不再进行重量差异检查；凡规定检查溶出度、释放度的片剂，不再进行崩解时限检查。

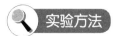 **实验器材**

1. 仪器 托盘天平、分析天平、单冲压片机、烘箱、研钵、烧杯、电炉、搪瓷盘、药筛（16目、80目、100目）、尼龙筛、量筒、试剂瓶、滴管、洗耳球、移液管、容量瓶、片剂硬度测定仪、崩解度测定仪、脆碎度检查仪、溶出度测定仪、紫外-可见分光光度计、石英比色皿、温度计、擦镜纸、微孔滤膜、镊子、吹风机等。

2. 材料 对乙酰氨基酚、阿司匹林、淀粉、聚山梨酯80、酒石酸、硬脂酸镁、滑石粉、乙醇、蒸馏水等。

实验方法

（一）对乙酰氨基酚片的制备

【处方】

对乙酰氨基酚	20g
淀粉	15g
聚山梨酯80	0.5g
淀粉浆（15%）	适量
硬脂酸镁	1%
95% 乙醇	适量
共制成 100 片	

【制法】

（1）取聚山梨酯80，溶于15ml乙醇中，加入淀粉，搅拌均匀，于70℃干燥，过100目筛，备用。

（2）取对乙酰氨基酚，置于研钵，研细，加入15%淀粉浆适量，制成软材。

（3）将软材挤压过16目筛，制成湿颗粒。

（4）将湿颗粒均匀置于方盘中，60℃干燥，干颗粒过16目筛整粒。

（5）将颗粒与（1）细粉混匀，加入硬脂酸镁，混匀，压片。

【性状】 本品为白色片剂。

【用途】 本品为解热镇痛药。用于感冒或感冒引起的发热，也可用于缓解轻至中度疼痛，如头痛、关节痛、偏头痛、牙痛、肌肉痛、神经痛、痛经等。

【注意事项】

（1）聚山梨酯80是表面活性剂，在该制剂中作为崩解辅助剂。

（2）淀粉浆用作黏合剂。淀粉浆的制备有两种方法。①煮浆法：取淀粉徐徐加入全量的水，不断搅匀，避免结块，加热并不断搅拌至沸，放冷即得。②冲浆法：取淀粉加少量冷水，搅匀，然后冲入一定量的沸水，不断搅拌，至成半透明糊状。此法适宜小量制备。

（3）淀粉浆以温浆加入为宜，容易分散均匀。淀粉浆的用量应适宜，以软材"手握成团、轻压即散"为度，保证制粒过程顺利进行。

（4）硬脂酸镁为疏水性润滑剂，用量不宜过大，否则影响片剂的崩解，一般用量为0.3%~1%。

（二）阿司匹林片的制备

【处方】

阿司匹林	30g

淀粉	3g
酒石酸	0.2g
淀粉浆（10%）	适量
干淀粉	4g
滑石粉	5%
蒸馏水	适量

共制成 300 片

【制法】

（1）取淀粉，置于烘箱，100~105℃干燥，使含水量在 8% 以下，制得干淀粉。

（2）取阿司匹林，置于研钵，研细，过 80 目筛。

（3）取酒石酸，溶于 50ml 蒸馏水中，煮沸，加到 5g 淀粉中，搅拌，制成 10% 淀粉浆。

（4）将阿司匹林细粉与淀粉混匀，加入适量淀粉浆制成软材，过 16 目筛，制成湿颗粒。

（5）湿颗粒于 40~50℃干燥，干颗粒过 16 目筛整粒，将此颗粒与干淀粉、滑石粉混匀，压片，即得。

【性状】本品为白色片剂。

【用途】解热镇痛药。主要用于发热、疼痛及类风湿关节炎等。

【注意事项】

（1）本品采用湿法制粒压片，阿司匹林在湿热条件下易水解成水杨酸和醋酸，增加对胃肠道黏膜的刺激性，故在淀粉浆中加入酒石酸，可减少阿司匹林的水解。

（2）金属离子可催化阿司匹林的水解，过筛时宜用尼龙筛网，并防止其变为红色。

（3）阿司匹林对热也不稳定，颗粒干燥温度应控制在 60℃以下。

（4）硬脂酸镁能促进阿司匹林的水解，故用滑石粉做润滑剂。

（三）片剂的质量检查

【性状】片剂应完整光洁，色泽均匀，有适宜的硬度。

【硬度】采用片剂硬度测定仪测定片剂硬度。一般能承受 40~60N 的压力即认为硬度适宜。

【脆碎度】取片剂适量（片重为 0.65g 及以下者，取若干片使其总重量约为 6.5g；片重大于 0.65g 者取 10 片），用吹风机吹去脱落的粉末，精密称重，置圆筒中，转动 100 次。取出，同法除去粉末，精密称重，减失的重量不得超过 1%。如减失重量超过 1% 时，应复验 2 次，3 次的平均减失重量不得超过 1%，并不得检出断裂、龟裂及粉碎的片。

【重量差异】取片剂 20 片，精密称定各片的重量，并计算出总重量和平均片重。每片重量与平均片重相比较，超出重量差异限度（平均片重小于 0.3g 者 ±7.5%，平均片重 0.3g 以上者 ±5.0%）的药片不得多于 2 片，并不得有 1 片超出限度一倍。

【崩解时限】取片剂 6 片，分别置于吊篮的玻璃管中进行检查，应在 15 分钟内全部崩解，如有 1 片不能完全溶散，应另取 6 片复试，均应符合规定。

【溶出度】取对乙酰氨基酚片 6 片，以稀盐酸 24ml 加水至 1000ml 为溶出介质，转速为每分钟 100 转，依法操作，经 30 分钟时，取溶液滤过，精密量取滤液适量，用 0.04% 氢氧化钠溶液稀释成每 1ml 中含对乙酰氨基酚 5~10μg 的溶液，照紫外－可见分光光度法在 257nm 的波长处测定吸光度，按 $C_8H_9NO_2$ 的吸收系数（$E_{1cm}^{1\%}$）为 715 计算每片溶出量，限度为标示量的 80%，应符合规定。

在溶出度测定时应注意：①转篮旋转时要求摆动幅度不得超过 ±1.0mm；②每只溶出杯里的介质温差不超过 0.5℃；③介质应脱气处理后使用，加入溶出杯中介质的体积误差率不大于 1%；④应在仪器开启的情况下取样，取样时，自取样至过滤应在 30 秒内完成。

实验结果与讨论

1. 结果 将对乙酰氨基酚片、阿司匹林片的质量检查结果填于表 8-1。

表 8-1 片剂质量检查结果

制剂	对乙酰氨基酚片	阿司匹林片
性状		
硬度		
脆碎度		
重量差异		
崩解时限		
溶出度		——

2. 讨论

（1）观察片剂外观性状，是否有裂片、松片等现象，分析原因。

（2）淀粉浆作为黏合剂，对片剂的崩解时限、溶出度有什么影响？

 思考题

1. 在制备片剂时，为什么要将原辅料制成颗粒后再压片？

2. 用于压片的颗粒与颗粒剂的颗粒有什么区别？

3. 片剂崩解剂的作用机制有哪些？

4. 对于湿热不稳定的药物，在进行片剂处方设计时，应注意哪些问题？

5. 如果要将制得的阿司匹林颗粒装入硬胶囊制成胶囊剂，应选择什么型号空胶囊？填装时需要注意哪些事项？

（韩　丽）

Lab. 8 Preparation and Quality Inspection of Tablets

 Experimental Objectives

1. To master the preparation methods of wet granulation techniques for tablets.

2. To be familiar with quality inspection methods of tablets, such as weight variation, hardness, friability, disintegration, dissolution, etc.

3. To understand the structure and working principle of tablet machine.

 Experimental Principles

Tablets are solid dosage forms made of drugs and suitable pharmaceutical excipients, usually in round or special tablet shape. Oral tablets include conventional tablets, sugar-coated tablets, film coated tablets, enteric coated tablets, chewable tablets, dispersible tablets, effervescent tablets, orally disintegrating tablets or orally dissolving tablets, sustained release tablets, controlled release tablets, multilayer tablets, and so on. Tablets used in the oral cavity include sublingual tablets, lozenges and buccaladhesive tablets, while solution tablets, vaginal tablets and vaginal effervescent tablets are usually applied externally. Tablets are one of the most widely used dosage forms in modern medicine.

According to their functions, the excipients of tablets can be divided into diluents, absorbents, wetting agents, binders, disintegrants, anti-adherents, glidants and lubricants, etc. Commonly used diluents include starch, powdered sugar, dextrin, lactose, compressible starch, microcrystalline cellulose, etc. Absorbents include calcium sulfate, calcium hydrogen phosphate. Wetting agents include water and ethanol. Binders include starch paste, cellulose derivatives, povidone, polyethylene glycol, gelatin, sucrose solution, etc. Disintegrants include dry starch, sodium starch glycolate, low-substituted hydroxypropyl cellulose, croscarmellose sodium, cross-linking povidone, effervescent disintegrants, etc. Lubricants include magnesium stearate, aerosil, talc, hydrogenated vegetable oil, sodium or magnesium lauryl sulfate, etc. Colorants and flavoring agents are also used as excipients of tablet as well.

The preparation methods of tablets can be divided into three types: wet granulation compression, dry granulation compression and direct compression of powers. The wet granulation compression method is suitable for most drugs except for those unstable to humidity and heat. The process is as follows.

Pulverizing → sieving → mixing → making soft materials → granulating → drying →sieving → final blending → compressing → (coating) → packaging

Methods for granulation include extrusion granulation, high-speed stirring granulation, fluidized bed granulation, spray granulation, etc. Extrusion granulation is usually used in the laboratory.

Notes for the preparation of tablets are as follows: ① Raw materials and excipients should be well mixed. ② Granulation and compression are the key processes for preparations of tablets. The shape, size, water content and compression characteristics of granules will affect the progress of compressing and qualities of obtained tablets. The tablet should have suitable hardness to meet the requirements for appearance and disintegration. ③ Drugs that are volatile or easily decomposed by heat should be protected from loss during the process. ④ Pressure should be moderate to ensure a certain hardness of tablets. ⑤ Sugar or film coating can be used for tablets with unpleasant odor, irritant, deliquescent or light-sensitive drugs. Enteric coating tablets is recommended for drugs which are easily destroyed by gastric juice or required to be released in the intestine.

The inspects of tablets include description, weight variation, hardness, friability, disintegration time, content uniformity, dissolution, release rate, etc. According to the requirements of the *Chinese Pharmacopoeia*, the weight viariation check is generally not performed for tablets that are required to check the content uniformity. Disintegration is no longer required for tablets that require dissolution and release rate.

 Equipments and Materials

1. Equipments   Counter balance, analytical balance, single-punch press, drying oven, mortar and pestle, beaker, electric furnace, enamel dish, stainless steel sieve(16 mesh, 80 mesh, 100 mesh), nylon sieve, measuring cylinder, reagent bottle, dropper, rubber suction bulb, pipette, volumetric flask, tablet hardness tester, disintegration determination apparatus, fragility tester, dissolution test apparatus, ultraviolet-visible spectrophotometer, quartz cuvette, thermometer, lens paper, microporous membrane, tweezers, hair dryer, etc.

2. Materials   Acetaminophen, aspirin, starch, polysorbate 80, tartaric acid, magnesium stearate, talcum powder, ethanol, distilled water, etc.

 Experimental Methods

I. Preparation of Acetaminophen Tablets
【Formula】

Acetaminophen	20g
Starch	15g
Polysorbate 80	0.5g
Starch paste (15%)	q.s.
Magnesium stearate	1%
95% Ethanol	q.s.

Make to 100 tablets

【Procedure】

(1) Dissolve polysorbate 80 in 15ml ethanol. Add starch, stir well, dry at 70℃, then pass through a 100 mesh sieve.

(2) Put acetaminophen in a motor, pulverize to fine power, add starch paste to make it into soft materials.

(3) Press soft materials through a 16-mesh sieve to make wet granules.

(4) Place wet granules in a square dish, dry at 60℃, sift through a 16 mesh.

(5) Mix granules with (1), add magnesium stearate, mix thoroughly, make into 100 tablets.

【Description】White tablets.

【Application】Antipyretic and analgesic. Commonly applied for colds or fever caused by cold, also for relieving pain, such as headache, joint pain, migraine, toothache, muscle pain, neuralgia, dysmenorrhea, etc.

【Notes】

(1) Polysorbate 80 is a surfactant that acts as a disintegration aid in this formulation.

(2) Starch paste is used as binder, the preparation of it is as follows.

① Boiling method: Add starch slowly into the full amount of water. Keep stirring to avoid caking until boiling, and then cool it. ② Flushing method: Take starch and add a small amount cold water, mix well, then add a certain amount of boiling water, continue to stir until it becomes translucent paste. This method is suitable for small amount preparation.

(3) The starch paste should be added in a warm state to facilitate dispersion, and an appropriate amount of paste should be used to make the soft material "holding into lumps, pressure lightly to disperse".

(4) Magnesium stearate is a hydrophobic lubricant, the amount should not be too large, otherwise it will affect the disintegration of tablets. General content is 0.3% to 1%.

II. Preparation of aspirin Tablets

【Formula】

aspirin	30g
Starch	3g
Tartaric acid	0.2g
Starch paste (10%)	q.s.
Dry starch	4g
Talcum powder	5%
Distilled water	q.s.

Make to 300 tablets

【Procedure】

(1) Put starch in an oven, dry at 100~105℃ to keep water content below 8%.

(2) Pulverize aspirin to fine power, pass through a 80 mesh sieve.

(3) Dissolve tartaric acid in 50ml distilled water, boil, add to 5g starch, stir well to make 10% starch paste.

(4) Mix aspirin powder with starch, make soft materials with a proper amount of starch paste, pass through of a 16 mesh sieve to get the wet granules.

(5) Dry granules at 40~50℃, sieve through 16 mesh, add dry starch and talcum powder, mix uniformly, compress into 300 tablets.

【Description】White tablets.

【Application】Antipyretic analgesic. It is mainly used for fever, pain and rheumatoid arthritis.

【Notes】

(1) Under the hot and humid condition, aspirin is easily hydrolyzed into salicylic acid and acetic, which can increase the irritation to the gastrointestinal mucosa. Therefore adding tartaric acid to starch paste can effectively prevent the hydrolysis of aspirin.

(2) Metal ions can accelerate the hydrolysis of aspirin. Nylon mesh should be used when sieving to

prevent the drug from turning red.

(3) The drying temperature should be controlled under 60℃ to ensure the stability of aspirin.

(4) Magnesium stearate can fasten the hydrolyzation of aspirin, so talcum powder is used as a lubricant.

III. Quality Inspection of Tablets

【Description】Tablets should be complete, bright and clean with uniform color and suitable hardness.

【Hardness】Inspect with tablet hardness tester. The suitable hardness is generally between 40~60N.

【Friability】Choose a proper amount of tablets (if the weight of tablets is 0.65g or less, take several tablets to make the total weight about 6.5g; if the weight of tablets is more than 0.65g, take 10 tablets), blow off the fallen powder with a hair dryer, weigh it accurately, put it in the cylinder, and rotate it 100 times. Take out, remove the powder with the same method, weigh accurately, and the weight lost shall not exceed 1%. If the weight loss is more than 1%, it shall be retested twice, and the average weight loss of three times shall not be more than 1%. The broken, cracked and smashed pieces shall not be detected.

【Weight Variation】Take 20 tablets, weigh each tablet precisely, and calculate the total weight and average tablet weight. When the weight of each tablet is compared with the average tablet weight, no more than 2 tablets shall exceed the weight variation limit (± 7.5% for tablets with an average tablet weight of less than 0.3g, and ± 5.0% for tablets with an average tablet weight of more than 0.3g), and no more than 1 tablet shall exceed the limit by one time.

【Disintegration】Take 6 tablets and place one tablet in each of the six tubes of the hanging basket and start the apparatus. All tablets should disintegrate completely within 15 minutes. If one tablet fail to meet the requirement of test, repeat the operation with another 6 tablets. All of which should meet the requirements.

【Dissolution】Add 24ml diluted hydrochloric acid in water to 1000ml as the dissolution medium. Take 6 acetaminophen tablets. Rotate the paddle at 100rpm. Withdraw the solution at 30 minutes, filter, dilute it with 0.04% sodium hydroxide solution to form a solution containing 5~10μg paracetamol per 1ml. Measure the absorbance of the solution at 257nm by UV-vis spectrophotometer. According to the absorption coefficient ($E_{1cm}^{1\%}$) of $C_8H_9NO_2$ (715), calculate the dissolution amount of each tablet. The limit is 80% of the labeled amount, the dissolution rate should meet the requirement.

【Notes】

(1) During the measurement of dissolution, the swing range of the rotating basket shall not exceed ± 1.0mm.

(2) The temperature difference of medium in each dissolving cup shall not exceed 0.5℃.

(3) The medium shall be used after degassing treatment, and the volume error rate of medium added into the dissolution cup shall not be greater than 1%.

(4) The sample shall be taken when the instrument is on, and the sampling shall be completed within 30 seconds from sampling to filtering.

Results and Discussions

1. Results Fill the quality inspection results of acetaminophen tablets and aspirin tablets in the Table 8-1.

Table 8–1 The quality inspection results of tablets

Preparation	Acetaminophen tablets	Aspirin tablets
Description		
Hardness		
Friability		
Weight variation		
Disintegration		
Dissolution		

2. Discussions

(1) Observe the appearance of tablets, whether there are cracks, loose ones, and analyze the reasons.

(2) What are the effects of starch paste on the disintegration and dissolution of tablets?

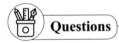 **Questions**

1. For most tablets, why should the raw materials and excipients be granulated before compression?

2. What are the difference between particles used for tablets and granules?

3. What are the action mechanisms of disintegrant?

4. When designing a tablet formulation, what should be paid attention to for drugs unstable in wet and hot environment?

5. Which kind of empty capsules should be selected if the acetylsalicylic acid granules are to be put into hard capsules? What should be taken into consideration while filling?

PPT

实验九 滴丸剂的制备及质量检查

实验目的

1. **掌握** 滴丸剂成型的原理及基本操作。
2. **熟悉** 滴丸剂的质量检查方法。

实验原理

滴丸系指固态或液态药物与适宜的基质加热熔融后，滴入不相混溶的冷凝液中，由于表面张力的作用使液滴收缩冷凝而成的球状制剂。

滴丸的基质有水溶性与非水溶性两大类，常用的水溶性基质有聚乙二醇（PEG）类，以 PEG 4000 或 PEG 6000 为常用，其熔点低（55~60℃），毒性小，化学性质稳定（在 100℃ 以上分解），能与多数药物配伍，具有良好的水溶性，能使难溶性药物以分子状态分散于载体中。在溶剂蒸发过程中，黏度逐渐增大，可阻止药物分子聚集。常用的非水溶性载体有虫蜡、硬脂酸、单硬脂酸甘油酯等，可使药物缓慢释放，也可用于水溶性载体中以调节熔点。

滴丸的制备工艺为：

药物 + 基质→熔融→滴制（保温）→冷却→洗丸→干燥→质检→包装

实验器材

1. **仪器** 天平、蒸发皿、恒温水浴锅、滴丸装置、胶头滴管、温度计、滤纸、脱脂棉、玻璃棒等。
2. **材料** 盐酸小檗碱、聚乙二醇 6000、苏合香、冰片、液状石蜡等。

实验方法

（一）盐酸小檗碱滴丸的制备

【处方】

盐酸小檗碱	0.1g
聚乙二醇 6000	10g
蒸馏水	适量

【制法】将盐酸小檗碱置于蒸发皿中，加少量蒸馏水加热使分散，加入聚乙二醇 6000 至熔化，搅匀，装入滴丸装置中，85℃ 保温，滴入事先冷却的液状石蜡冷却剂中，冷凝成丸。

滴制完毕，将滴丸继续留在冷却剂中，使其充分冷却，取出滴丸，摊在滤纸上，吸去滴丸表面的液状石蜡（必要时可用乙醇洗涤），自然干燥，即得。

【性状】本品为黄色圆球形滴丸。

62

【用途】具有抗菌作用，用于治疗痢疾。

【注意事项】滴丸滴制时熔融药液的温度应不低于 80℃，否则药液在滴口处易凝固，难以滴下，同时应尽可能保持恒温，使滴丸大小均匀。

（二）苏冰滴丸的制备

【处方】

苏合香	1.0g
冰片	2.0g
聚乙二醇 6000	7.0g

【制法】将聚乙二醇 6000 置蒸发皿中，水浴加热至全部熔融，加入苏合香、冰片，搅拌至溶解，90℃保温，滴入 10~15℃ 的液状石蜡中，冷凝成丸，取出滴丸，摊在纸上，吸去滴丸表面的液状石蜡，即得。

【性状】本品为淡黄色滴丸，气芳香，味辛、苦。

【用途】芳香开窍，理气止痛。用于冠心病导致的胸闷、心绞痛等。

【注意事项】冰片与基质混匀前应研细，必要时可加少许乙醇共研，以保证滴丸的光滑度。

（三）滴丸的质量检查

【重量差异】照 2020 年版《中国药典》重量差异检查法检查。取滴丸 20 丸，精密称定总重量，求得平均丸重后，再分别精密称定每丸的重量。每丸重量与平均丸重相比较，超出限度（0.03g以下或 0.03g 为 ±15%，0.03g 以 上 至 0.3g 为 ±12%，0.3g 以 上 至 0.1g 为 ±10%，0.3g 以 上 为 ±7.5%）的不得多于 2 丸，并不得有 1 粒超出限度一倍。

【溶散时限】照 2020 年版《中国药典》溶散时限检查法检查。取滴丸 6 粒，分别置于吊篮的玻璃管中，加挡板，启动崩解仪进行检查，应在 30 分钟内全部溶散，如有 1 粒不能完全溶散，应另取 6 粒复试，均应符合规定。

实验结果与讨论

1. 结果　将盐酸小檗碱滴丸、苏冰滴丸的质量检查结果填入表 9-1。

表 9-1　盐酸小檗碱滴丸、苏冰滴丸的检查结果

制剂	盐酸小檗碱滴丸	苏冰滴丸
性状		
重量差异		
溶散时限		

2. 讨论　操作中哪些因素会影响实验结果？

思考题

1. 滴丸制备中应注意哪些问题？怎样进行质量控制？

2. 如何选择滴丸的基质与冷凝液？

3. 滴丸速效作用机制有哪些？

Lab. 9 | Preparation and Quality Inspection of Dripping Pills

Experimental Objectives

1. To master the principle and basic operation of dripping pills formation.
2. To be familiar with the quality inspection methods of dripping pills.

Experimental Principles

Dripping pills refers to a spherical preparation in which a solid or liquid drug is heated and melted with suitable excipients, and then dripped into an immiscible condensate, which shrinks and condenses due to the effect of surface tension.

The matrix of dripping pills has two types: water-soluble and water-insoluble. The commonly used water-soluble matrix is polyethylene glycol (PEG). PEG 4000 or PEG 6000 is widely used. It has a low melting point (55~60℃), low toxicity and stable chemical properties (decomposed above 100℃), can be compatible with most drugs, has good water solubility, and can make poorly soluble drugs dispersed in the carrier in a molecular state. During the evaporation of the solvent, the viscosity gradually increases, which prevents the drug molecules from aggregating. Common water-insoluble carriers include insect wax, stearic acid, glycerin monostearate, etc., which can slowly release the drug, and can also be used in water-soluble carriers to adjust the melting point.

The preparation process of dripping pills:

Drug + matrix → melting → drop (heat preservation) → cooling → washing pills → drying → quality inspection → package

Equipments and Materials

1. Equipments Electronic scales, evaporation dish, constant temperature water bath kettle, pill dropping device, plastic dropper, thermometer, filter paper, absorbent cotton, glass rod, etc.

2. Materials Berberine hydrochloride, polyethylene glycol 6000, styrax, borneol, liquid paraffin, etc.

Experimental Methods

I. Preparation of Berberine Hydrochloride Dripping Pills

【Formula】

Berberine hydrochloride	0.1g
PEG 6000	10g

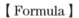

Distilled water　　　　　　　　　　　q.s.

【Procedure】Place berberine hydrochloride in an evaporating dish, and heat it up with a little distilled water to disperse it. Add PEG 6000 to melt, stir well, and then put it into the drop pill device. Keep the temperature at 85℃. After a period of heat preservation, the drug is dropped into a pre-cooled liquid paraffin coolant and condensed into pellets.

After the dripping is completed, leave the dropping pills in the coolant and let them cool down sufficiently. Take out the dripping pills, spread them on filter paper, suck off the liquid paraffin on the dripping pills surface (wash with ethanol if necessary), and dry it.

【Description】Berberine hydrochloride dropping pills are yellow spherical dripping pills.

【Application】Berberine hydrochloride dropping pills have antibacterial effect and are used to treat dysentery.

【Notes】The temperature of the molten medicinal solution should not be lower than 80℃ during dripping. Otherwise, the medicinal solution is easy to solidify at the mouth of the drip and difficult to drip. At the same time, it should be kept as constant as possible to make the size of the dripping pills uniform.

II. Preparation of Subing Dripping Pills

【Formula】

Styrax　　　　　　　　　　　　　　1.0g

Borneol　　　　　　　　　　　　　　2.0g

PEG 6000　　　　　　　　　　　　　7.0g

【Procedure】Place PEG 6000 in an evaporation dish, heat it in a water bath until it melts completely, add styrax and borneol, stir it until it dissolves, keep it at 90℃, drip it into liquid paraffin at 10℃ to 15℃, and condense it into pellets. Take out the dripping pills, spread it on paper, and suck off the liquid paraffin on the surface of the dripping pills.

【Description】Subing dripping pills are pale yellow dripping pills, which are fragrant, taste bitter.

【Application】Fragrant, invigorating, regulating qi and relieving pain. Subing dripping pills are used for chest tightness and angina pectoris caused by coronary heart disease.

【Notes】Before mixing borneol and matrix, grind them fine, if necessary, add a little ethanol to grind them together to ensure the smoothness of the dripping pills.

III. Quality Inspection of Dripping Pills

【Weight variation】According to the *Chinese Pharmacopoeia* (2020) "Weight variation" inspection method for inspection. Take 20 drops of pills and accurately weigh the total weight. After obtaining the average weight of the pills, weigh the weight of each pellet separately. Comparing the weight of each pill with the average pill weight, exceeding the limit (0.03g or less or 0.03g is "±15%", 0.03g or more and 0.3g is "±12%", 0.3g or more and 0.1g is "±10%", and 0.3g or more is "±7.5%") of no more than 2 pills, and no more than 1 pill would exceed the limit double.

【Dissolution time limit】According to *Chinese Pharmacopoeia* (2020) "Dissolution time limit inspection method". Take 6 dripping pills, put them in the glass tube of the hanging basket, add the baffle plate, start the disintegrating instrument for inspection, and dissolve them all within 30 minutes. If one of them can not be completely dissolved, another 6 pills should be taken for the second test, all of the 6 pills should meet the requirements.

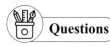 **Results and Discussion**

1. Results   The quality inspection results of berberine hydrochloride dropping pills and Subing dripping pills are shown in the Table 9–1.

Table 9–1   Test results of berberine hydrochloride dripping pills and Subing dripping pills

Preparation	Berberine hydrochloride dripping pills	Subing dripping pills
Description		
Weight variation		
Dissolution time limit		

2. Discussions   What factors in the operation will affect the experimental results?

Questions

1. What should be paid attention to in the preparation of dripping pills? How to control the quality?
2. How to choose the substrate and condensate of dripping pills?
3. What are the quick-acting mechanisms of dripping pills?

实验十　栓剂的制备及置换价的测定

 实验目的

1．**掌握**　热熔法制备栓剂的流程及操作要点。
2．**熟悉**　置换价测定方法及应用，栓剂质量评价的方法。

实验原理

栓剂是指药物与适宜基质制成的专供腔道给药的固体制剂，常温下为固体，纳入腔道后应能迅速软化熔融或溶解。根据栓剂中药物吸收特点，栓剂可以发挥局部作用和全身作用。临床常用的栓剂主要有直肠栓和阴道栓，此外还有尿道栓、耳用栓、鼻用栓等。根据使用腔道不同，栓剂常制成鱼雷形、圆锥形、圆柱形、球形、卵形、鸭嘴形等。

栓剂主要由药物和基质组成，根据需要可加入适量附加剂。药物要求能溶于基质或均匀混悬于基质中，除另有规定外，应为 100 目以上的粉末。基质可分为油脂性基质与水溶性基质两类。油脂类基质常用可可豆脂、半合成或全合成脂肪酸甘油酯等。水溶性基质常用品种有甘油明胶、聚乙二醇、泊洛沙姆、聚氧乙烯单硬脂酸酯类。栓剂根据需要可加入硬化剂、增稠剂、吸收促进剂、抗氧剂和防腐剂等。

栓剂的制备方法主要有热熔法、冷压法和搓捏法三种，其中热熔法最为常用。热熔法制备栓剂的工艺流程为：

基质→融化→药物混合→注入栓模→冷却→削平→脱模→质检→包装

在制备过程中，为了使栓剂冷却后易于从栓模中推出，在注入前应涂适量润滑剂。润滑剂的性质应该与基质性质相反，水溶性基质涂油溶性润滑剂，如液状石蜡或植物油等；油溶性基质涂水溶性润滑剂，如软皂乙醇液（软皂、甘油各 1 份及 90% 乙醇 5 份混合而成）。

置换价（displacement value，DV）指主药的重量与同体积基质重量的比值。通常情况下，同一模型容积是相同的，但制成的栓剂质量则随基质与药物密度的不同而有差异，为了确定不同栓剂基质用量，保证药物剂量的准确，常需测定药物的置换价。因此，对于药物与基质的密度相差较大及药物含量较高的栓剂，置换价的测定显得尤为重要。可用公式（10-1）计算药物对基质的置换价。

$$DV=\frac{W}{G-(M-W)} \tag{10-1}$$

式中，W 为每枚栓剂中主药的重量；G 为每枚纯基质栓剂的重量；M 为每枚含药栓剂的重量。

根据式（10-1）求得的置换价，求算出每枚栓剂中应投料的基质质量（x）为：

$$x=G-\frac{y}{DV} \tag{10-2}$$

式中，y 为处方中药物的剂量。

2020 年版《中国药典》规定，栓剂在生产和贮存期间应符合以下有关规定：外形完整光滑；

纳入腔道后应无刺激性，应能融化、软化或溶化，并与分泌液混合，逐渐释放出药物，产生局部或全身治疗作用；应有适宜的硬度，以免在包装或贮存时变形。

实验器材

1. **仪器** 栓剂融变时限测定仪、电子天平、栓模、烧杯、水浴锅、玻璃棒、量筒等。
2. **材料** 乙酰水杨酸、半合成脂肪酸甘油酯、聚氧乙烯（40）单硬脂酸酯、甘油、硬脂酸、氢氧化钠、液状石蜡、软皂、乙醇、蒸馏水等。

实验方法

（一）置换价的测定

以乙酰水杨酸为模型药物，用半合成脂肪酸甘油酯为基质进行置换价测定。

1. 纯基质栓的制备

【处方】

半合成脂肪酸甘油酯　　　　　　　　　　10g

【制法】取半合成脂肪酸甘油酯10g，置干燥烧杯中，于水浴上加热搅拌使熔化，待基质呈黏稠状态时，倾入预先涂有软皂乙醇液的栓模中，冷却至完全固化，削去栓模上溢出部分，脱模，得到完整的纯基质栓数枚，称重，每枚纯基质的平均重量为 G（g）。

2. 含药栓（乙酰水杨酸栓）的制备

【处方】

半合成脂肪酸甘油酯　　　　　　　　　　6g

乙酰水杨酸　　　　　　　　　　　　　　3g

【制法】取半合成脂肪酸甘油酯6g，置干燥烧杯中，于水浴上加热搅拌使熔化；称取乙酰水杨酸粉末（100目）3g，分次加入已熔化的基质中，搅拌使药物分散均匀，待混合物呈黏稠状态时，倾入预先涂有软皂乙醇液的栓模中，冷却至完全固化，削去栓模上溢出部分，脱模，得到完整的含药栓数枚，称重，每枚含药栓的平均质量为 M（g），每枚栓剂含药量 $W=M \cdot X\%$，$X\%$ 为栓剂含药百分量。

【计算】将上述得到的 G、M、W 代入式（10-1），计算乙酰水杨酸对半合成脂肪酸甘油酯的置换价。

（二）甘油栓的制备

【处方】

甘油	10g
硬脂酸	0.8g
氢氧化钠	0.12g
蒸馏水	1.4ml

【制法】称取甘油置烧杯中，水浴加热（100℃），加入研细的硬脂酸、氢氧化钠和水，不断搅拌使其溶解，继续于85~95℃保温至澄清，倾入预先涂有液状石蜡的栓模中，冷却至完全固化，削去栓模上溢出部分，脱模，质检，包装，即得。

【性状】本品为白色或几乎无色的透明或半透明栓。

【用途】润滑性泻药。

【注意事项】

（1）制备甘油栓时，水浴要保持沸腾，硬脂酸细粉应少量分次加入，与碱充分反应后，直至溶液澄明才能停止加热；产生的二氧化碳须除尽，否则所得的栓剂内含有气泡，影响美观。

（2）注模前应将栓模预热，注模后缓缓冷却，冷却太快会影响栓剂质量。

（三）栓剂的质量检查

【外观】检查上述制备的栓剂外观是否完整，表面亮度是否一致，有无斑点和气泡。将栓剂纵向剖开，观察药物分散是否均匀。

【重量差异】照 2020 年版《中国药典》栓剂项下相关规定进行。取栓剂 10 粒，精密称定总重量，计算平均重量，再分别精密称定各粒的重量。每粒重量与平均粒重相比较，超出重量差异限度（平均粒重 1.0g 及 1.0g 以下者 ±10%，1.0g 以上至 3.0g 者 ±7.5%，3.0g 以上者 ±5.0%）的不得多于 1 粒，并不得超出限度一倍。

【融变时限】照 2020 年版《中国药典》融变时限检查法检查。取栓剂 3 粒，在室温放置 1 小时后，按融变时限检查的装置和方法进行检查。脂肪性基质的栓剂应在 30 分钟内全部融化、软化或触压时无硬心；水溶性栓剂应在 60 分钟内全部溶解。

实验结果与讨论

1. 根据置换价计算公式计算乙酰水杨酸对半合成脂肪酸甘油酯的置换价。
2. 将栓剂的各项质量检查结果记录于表 10-1。

表 10-1　栓剂质量检查结果

名称	外观	重量 /g	重量差异	融变时限 /min
乙酰水杨酸栓				
甘油栓				

3. 比较各组实验制品的外观、形状，观察是否有气泡，分析原因。
4. 甘油栓的制备原理是什么？操作时应注意哪些要点？

思考题

1. 热熔法制备栓剂时，注模应注意哪些问题？
2. 在栓剂制备过程中，如何保证药物与基质混合均匀？
3. 栓剂在选择基质时主要考虑哪些因素？

（颜　红）

Lab. 10 Preparation of Suppositories and Determination of Displacement Value

 Experimental Objectives

1. To master the process and key points of hot melt suppository preparation.

2. To be familiar with the measurement method and application of displacement value, the evaluation method of suppository quality.

 Experimental Principles

Suppositories are solid preparations made by incorporating drug substances in suitable bases, intended for administration to cavities. At room temperature, they are solid but can soften, melt or dissolve rapidly after being inserted into the cavity. According to different absorption characteristics of drugs in suppositories, suppositories can exert local and systemic effect. Rectal suppositories and vaginal suppositories are commonly used in clinic practice, in addition, there are urethral suppositories, ear suppositories, nasal suppositories, etc. Based on the different cavities they are intended to be applied to, suppositories are usually cylindrical, conical, spherical, oval or "torpedo" shaped.

Suppositories are mainly composed of drugs and bases, if necessary with appropriate additives. The drugs are required to be soluble or uniformly suspended in bases and, unless otherwise specified, should be in powder form of more than 100-mesh. Bases are classified into oleaginous and water-soluble bases. Oleaginous bases include cocoa butter, semi-synthetic or fully-synthetic fatty glycerides, etc, while common varieties of water-soluble bases include glycerolgelatin, polyethylene glycol, poloxamers and polyoxyethylene stearate. Hardening agents, thickening agents, absorption promoters, antioxidants, preservatives, etc. may be added in suppositories as required.

Suppositories are mainly prepared by hot melt, cold pressing and kneading, of which hot melt is the most commonly used method. The process of hot melt preparation is shown as follows:

Bases → melting → drug mixing → injection into mold → cooling → leveling → demolding → quality inspection → packaging

During the preparation process, in order to make it easier to remove the suppository from the mold after cooling, an appropriate amount of lubricant should be applied before injection. The nature of the lubricant should be opposite to that of bases. That is to say, water-soluble bases should be coated with an oil-soluble lubricant, such as liquid paraffin or vegetable oil, while oil-soluble bases should be coated with water-soluble lubricant, such as soft soap ethanol solution (mixed in the following proportions: 1 part soft soap, 1 part glycerol and 5 parts 90% ethanol).

Displacement value (DV) refers to the ratio of the weight of the main drugs to the weight of the same volume of bases. Under normal circumstances, the volume of the same model is equal, but the quality of the prepared suppository varies with the density of bases and drugs. It is necessary to determine displacement value in order to determine the base dosage of different suppositories and ensure the accuracy of drugs dosage. Therefore, for suppositories with large density differences between drugs and bases, or with high drug content, the determination of displacement value is particularly important. Formula 10–1 below can be used to calculate the displacement value of drugs to bases.

$$DV=\frac{W}{G-(M-W)} \tag{10-1}$$

Where, W is the weight of the main drug in each suppository; G is the weight of each pure suppository base and M is the weight of each suppository.

According to the displacement value obtained by the above formula, the base mass (x) in each suppository is calculated as follows:

$$x=G-\frac{y}{DV} \tag{10-2}$$

Where, y is the dosage of drugs in the prescription.

The *Chinese Pharmacopoeia* (2020) stipulates that suppositories should meet the following requirements during production, packaging and storage: they should look intact and smooth. Suppositories should be non-irritating and able to be melted, softened or dissolved when inserted into the cavity and be miscible with body fluid to release the drug substances gradually, thus exert local or systemic effect. They should also be appropriately hard to prevent deformation during packaging or storage.

 Equipments and Materials

1. Equipments   Disintegration tester, electronic balance, mold, beaker, water bath pan, glass rod, measuring cylinder, etc.

2. Materials   Acetylsalicylic acid, semi-synthetic fatty glycerides, polyoxyethylene (40) monostearate, glycerol, stearic acid, sodium hydroxide, liquid paraffin, soft soap, ethanol, distilled water, etc.

 Experimental Methods

I. Determination of Displacement Value

Acetylsalicylic acid is used as the model drug and semi-synthetic fatty glycerides as the base to determine displacement value.

1. Preparation of pure base suppository

【Formula】

Semi-synthetic fatty glycerides   10g

【Procedure】Put 10g of semi-synthetic fatty glycerides into a dry beaker, and place in a water bath and heat to melting point. When it is viscous, pour it into a mold pre-coated with soft soap ethanol solution. Allow it to cool down and completely solidify in following step, before trimming-off any excess material from the mold. The ultimate stages of the preparation include demolding to obtain a complete number of suppositories containing pure bases, and obtain the average mass of each suppositories - G(g).

2. Preparation of drug-containing suppositories (acetylsalicylic acid suppositories)

【Formula】

Semi-synthetic fatty glycerides	6g
Acetylsalicylic acid	3g

【Procedure】Place 6g of semisynthetic fatty glycerides into a dry beaker, and put in a water bath and heat to melting point. Next, weigh 3g of acetylsalicylic acid powder (100 mesh) and add it into the melted base in batches, stirring to disperse the drug evenly. When the mixture is viscous, pour it into a suppository mold pre-coated with soft soap ethanol solution, allow it to cool down and solidify before trimming-off any excess material from the mold. The final stages of the preparation include demolding to obtain several complete suppositories containing drugs, and get the average mass of each suppository containing drugs - M (g), the dosage of each suppository is $W = MX\%$, and $X\%$ is the percentage of each suppository containing drugs.

【Calculation】Substituting G, M and W obtained above into Formula 10–1, the displacement value of acetylsalicylic acid to semi-synthetic fatty glycerides is calculated.

II. Preparation of Glycerol Suppository

【Formula】

Glycerin	10g
Stearic acid	0.8g
Sodium hydroxide	0.12g
Distilled water	1.4ml

【Procedure】Put 10g of glycerin into a glass beaker, and place in a water bath and heat to 100℃. Then, add the ground stearic acid, sodium hydroxide and water, continuously stirring until the solution dissolves. The temperature of the mixture should then be lowered and kept at 85~95℃ until it clears. Once the mixture is translucent, pour it into a bolt mold, pre-coated with liquid paraffin, allow it to cool down and solidify before trimming-off any excess material from the mold. The final stages of the suppository preparation include demolding, quality inspection and packaging.

【Description】White or almost colorless transparent or translucent suppository.

【Application】Lubricant laxative.

【Notes】

(1) When preparing the glycerol suppository, the water bath should be kept boiling. Stearic acid fine powder should be added in small amounts and in batches. After fully reacting with sodium hydroxide, heat continuously until the solution becomes clear. The carbon dioxide produced must be removed completely, otherwise the suppository contains bubbles, which will affect the appearance.

(2) Preheat the suppository mold prior to, and slowly cool it after mold injection. Note that cooling too fast will affect the suppository quality.

III. Quality Inspection of the Suppositories

【Appearance】Check whether the suppository prepared above is complete in appearance, uniform in surface brightness, and free from spots and bubbles. Cut the suppository longitudinally to observe whether the drug is evenly dispersed.

【Weight Variation】Suppositories should comply with the relevant provisions under the Suppositories in the *Chinese Pharmacopoeia* (2020). Weigh accurately together 10 suppositories and calculate the average weight; then individually weigh each of the 10 suppositories. None of the individual weights should deviate from the average weight by more than the weight variation limit (if the average weight is 1.0g or less, the weigh variation shall not deviate from 10%; if the average weight is between 1.0g and 3.0g, the weight variation limit is 7.5%; if the weight is more than 3.0g, the limit is 5.0%) and none deviates from twice of the limit.

【Disintegration Test】Suppositories should comply with the requirements of disintegration test for suppositories in the *Chinese Pharmacopoeia* (2020). Take 3 suppositories and allow them to remain at room temperature for 1 hour before checking. Suppositories of fatty bases should be completely melted, softened or pressed (through to the core) within 30 minutes; water-soluble suppositories should dissolve completely within 60 minutes.

 Results and Discussions

1. Calculate the displacement value of acetylsalicylic acid to semi-synthetic fatty glycerides according to the formula.

2. Record the quality inspection results in the Table 10–1.

Table 10–1   Quality inspection results of suppositories

Name	Appearance	Weight/g	Weight Variation	Disintegration Test/min
Acetylsalicylic acid				
Glycerol suppositories				

3. Compare the appearance and shape of the experimental products of each group, observe whether there are bubbles, and analyze the reasons.

4. What is the preparation principle of glycerol suppositories? What key points should be paid attention to during preparation?

Questions

1. What should we notice when preparing suppositories by the hot melt method?

2. In the process of suppository preparation, how to ensure that the drugs and bases are mixed uniformly?

3. What are the main factors to consider when choosing the suppository bases?

实验十一　膜剂的制备

PPT

实验目的

1. **掌握**　实验室制备膜剂的方法和操作注意事项。
2. **熟悉**　膜剂常用成膜材料的性质和特点。

实验原理

膜剂系指原料药物与适宜的成膜材料经加工制成的膜状制剂。一般膜剂的厚度为0.05~0.2mm，面积依临床应用部位而有差别。膜剂的给药途径广，可供内服（如口服、口含、舌下），外用（如皮肤、黏膜），腔道用（如阴道），植入或眼用等。膜剂根据结构特点分为单层膜、多层膜、夹心膜等。

成膜材料的性能和质量对膜剂的成型工艺、质量及药效有重要影响。常用的成膜材料，天然高分子材料有明胶、阿拉伯胶、琼脂、淀粉、糊精等；合成高分子材料有聚乙烯醇（PVA）、聚乙烯吡咯烷酮（PVP）、乙烯–醋酸乙烯共聚物（EVA）及丙烯酸树脂类、聚乙烯醇缩乙醛等。最常用的成膜材料是PVA，一种由聚醋酸乙烯酯经醇解而成的结晶性高分子材料。PVA的性质主要由其分子量和醇解度决定，分子量越大，水溶性越差，但水溶液的黏度越大，成膜性能越好。国内常用的PVA型号为05–88和17–88两种规格，平均聚合度分别为500~600和1700~1800。前者聚合度小，则分子量小，水中溶解度大而黏度较小。后者分子量大，水中溶解度较小而黏度较大。这两种规格的醇解度均为88%，一般认为此时水溶性最好，在温水中能很快溶解。两者常以适当比例混合使用。

膜剂处方中除主药和成膜材料外，一般还需加入增塑剂、表面活性剂、填充剂、着色剂、矫味剂等附加剂，制备时需根据成膜材料性质加入适宜的脱膜剂，如以PVA为膜材时，脱膜剂可采用液状石蜡。

膜剂的制备一般采用涂膜法，工艺流程为：配制成膜材料浆液→加入药物、附加剂混匀→脱泡→涂膜→干燥、灭菌→脱膜→质检→分剂量→包装。

膜剂制备时常见的问题及产生的原因有：干燥温度太高或玻璃板等未洗净、未涂润滑剂导致药膜不易剥离；开始干燥温度太高会导致药膜表面有不均匀气泡；油的含量太高以及成膜材料选择不当使得药膜走油；固体成分含量太高使得药粉从药膜上"脱落"；增塑剂太少或太多会导致药膜太脆或太软；未经过滤或溶解的药物从浆液中析出结晶会导致药膜中有粗大颗粒；浆液久置、药物沉淀以及不溶性成分粒子太大导致药膜中药物含量不均匀。

实验器材

1. **仪器**　恒温水浴锅、研钵、玻璃板、量筒、烘箱、玻璃棒、托盘天平、烧杯等。
2. **材料**　甲硝唑、聚乙烯醇（17–88）、硝酸钾、甘油、羧甲基纤维素钠（CMC-Na）、聚山梨酯 80、糖精钠、蒸馏水等。

实验方法

（一）甲硝唑口腔溃疡膜的制备

【处方】

甲硝唑	0.3g
聚乙烯醇（17-88）	5g
甘油	0.3g
蒸馏水	50ml

【制法】取 PVA、甘油、蒸馏水，搅拌浸泡溶胀后于 90℃水浴上加热使溶解，趁热用 80 目筛网过滤，滤液放冷后加甲硝唑，搅拌使溶解，放置一定时间除气泡，然后倒在玻璃板（预先涂少量液状石蜡）上用刮板法制膜，于 80℃干燥后切成 1cm^2 的小片，包装即得。

【注意事项】

（1）PVA 在浸泡溶胀时应加盖，以免水分蒸发，难以充分溶胀。溶解后应趁热过滤，除去杂质，放冷后不易过滤。

（2）药物与胶浆混匀后应静置除去气泡，涂膜时不宜搅拌，以免形成气泡。除气泡后应及时制膜，久置后，药物易沉淀，使含量不均匀。

（二）硝酸钾牙用膜剂的制备

【处方】

硝酸钾	1.5g
羧甲基纤维素钠（CMC-Na）	3.0g
聚山梨酯 80	0.3g
甘油	0.3g
糖精钠	0.1g
蒸馏水	适量

【制法】取 CMC-Na 加蒸馏水 60ml 浸泡，放置过夜，次日于水浴上加热溶解，制成胶浆。另取甘油、聚山梨酯 80 混匀，加硝酸钾、糖精钠、蒸馏水 5ml，必要时加热溶解，在搅拌下倒入胶浆内，于 40℃保温除泡，制膜，80℃烘干，即得。

【注意事项】

（1）成膜材料 CMC-Na 在水中浸泡时间必须充分，保证充分溶胀；水浴溶解时温度不宜超过 40℃。

（2）硝酸钾应完全溶解于水中后再与胶浆混匀，且制膜后应立即烘干，以免硝酸钾析出结晶，造成药膜中有粗大结晶及药物含量不均匀。

实验结果与讨论

1. 将甲硝唑口腔溃疡膜、硝酸钾牙用膜剂的性状检查实验结果记录于表 11-1 中。

表 11-1　甲硝唑口腔溃疡膜、硝酸钾牙用膜剂的性状检查结果

名称	外观	厚度	色泽	气泡
甲硝唑口腔溃疡膜				
硝酸钾牙用膜剂				

2. 试根据实验结果分析聚乙烯醇（17-88）与羧甲基纤维素钠的成膜性能差异。

 思考题

1. 小量制备膜剂时，常用哪些成膜方法？其操作要点有哪些？
2. 膜剂处方中各种辅料的作用是什么？
3. 膜剂制备时，如何防止气泡的产生？

（孙 黎）

Lab. 11　Preparation of Films

 Experimental Objectives

1. To master the methods and operation notes of films preparation in laboratory.
2. To be familiar with the properties and characteristics of common-used film-forming materials.

 Experimental Principles

Film refers to a kind of membrane preparation which is made of drugs and suitable film-forming materials. Generally, the thickness of the general film is 0.05~0.2mm, and the area varies depending on the clinical application site. The administration route of the film is wide and can be used for oral administration (such as oral, buccal, sublingual), external use (such as skin, mucous membranes), cavity use (such as vagina), implantation or ophthalmic etc. According to the structural characteristics, the film can be divided into monolayer, multilayer, sandwich film, etc.

The performance and quality of film-forming materials have an important impact on the molding process, quality and efficacy of filming agents. Commonly used materials, the natural polymer materials include gelatin, gum arabic, agar, starch, dextrin, etc; the synthetic polymer materials include polyvinyl alcohol (PVA), polyvinyl pyrrolidone (PVP), ethylene-vinyl acetate copolymer (EVA), acrylic resins, polyvinyl acetal, etc. The most commonly used film-forming material is PVA, which is a crystalline polymer material formed by alcoholysis of polyvinyl acetate. The properties of PVA are mainly determined by its molecular weight and alcoholysis degree. The larger the molecular weight, the worse the water solubility, but the greater the viscosity of the aqueous solution, the better the film forming performance. The PVA models are two specifications of 05-88 and 17-88, with average polymerization degrees of 500 ~ 600 and 1700~1800 respectively. The former has small degree of polymerization, small molecular weight, high solubility in water and low viscosity. The latter has high molecular weight, low solubility and high viscosity. The alcoholysis degree of the two specifications is 88%. It is generally considered that the water solubility is the best at this time, and it can be quickly dissolved in warm water. They are often mixed in an appropriate proportion.

In addition to the main drug and film-forming materials, plasticizers, surfactants, fillers, colorants, flavor rectifiers and other additives should be added in the formulation of film-forming materials. Appropriate film removers should be added according to the properties of film-forming materials. For example, when PVA is used as film material, liquid paraffin can be used as the film-forming agent.

The preparation of film generally adopts the coating method, and the technological process is as follows: Preparing membrane material slurry → adding drugs and additives to mix well → defoaming → coating → drying and sterilization → stripping → quality inspection → dosage division → packaging.

Common problems and reasons for the preparation of the film agent are: The film is not easy to peel due to the high drying temperature or the unclean and uncoated glass plate; too high initial drying temperature will lead to uneven bubbles on the surface of the drug film, too high oil content and improper selection of film-forming materials will lead to oil removal of the drug film; too high content of solid components makes the powder "fall off" from the drug film; too little or too much plasticizer will cause the drug film to be too brittle or too soft; the separation and crystallization of unfiltered or dissolved drugs from the slurry will cause coarse particles in the drug film; the long-standing slurry, drug precipitation and too large insoluble constituent particles will cause uneven drug content in the drug film.

 Equipments and Materials

1. Equipments　Thermostatic water bath, mortar, glass plate, graduatedcylinde, oven, glass rod, pallet balance, beaker, etc.

2. Materials　Metronidazole, polyvinyl alcohol (17-88), potassium nitrate, glycerol, carboxymethylcellulose sodium (CMC-Na), polysorbate 80, saccharin sodium, distilled water, etc.

 Experimental Methods

Ⅰ. Preparation of Metronidazole Oral Ulcer Film

【Formula】

Metronidazole	0.3g
Polyvinyl alcohol (17-88)	5g
Glycerol	0.3g
Distilled water	50ml

【Procedure】Take PVA, glycerol and distilled water, stir them for soaking and swelling, heat them on a 90℃ water bath to dissolve them, filter them with 80 mesh screen while they are hot, cool the filtrate, add metronidazole, stir to dissolve and placed for a certain time to remove bubbles, then pour them on a glass plate (previously coated with a small amount of liquid paraffin) and make a pellicle by scraping plate method, dry them at 80℃ and cut them into small pieces of 1cm^2, then pack them.

【Notes】

(1) PVA should be covered when soaking and swelling to avoid water evaporation and full swelling. After dissolution, it should be filtered while hot to remove impurities, it is not easy to filter after cooling.

(2) After the drug and glue are mixed, the bubbles should be removed by standing, and the film should not be stirred to avoid bubbles. After removing the air bubbles, the film should be formed in time. After long-term storage, the drug is easy to precipitate and the content is uneven.

Ⅱ. Preparation of Potassium Nitrate Dental Film

【Formula】

Potassium nitrate	1.5g
Carboxymethylcellulose sodium (CMC-Na)	3.0g
Polysorbate 80	0.3g
Glycerol	0.3g
Saccharin sodium	0.1g
Distilled water	q.s.

【Procedure】Soak CMC-Na in 60ml distilled water, leave it overnight, heat and dissolve in a water bath the next day to make a mucilage. Add glycerol and polysorbate 80 and mix, add potassium nitrate, saccharin sodium, 5ml of distilled water, heat and dissolve if necessary, pour them into the mortar under mixing, heat and defoam at 40℃, make a film, and dry at 80℃.

【Notes】

(1) The CMC-Na must be immersed in water for a sufficient time to ensure sufficient swelling; the temperature should not exceed 40℃ when dissolving in water bath.

(2) Potassium nitrate should be completely dissolved in water before mixing, and it should be dried immediately after film formation, so as to avoid crystallization of potassium nitrate, resulting in coarse crystallization and uneven drug content in the film.

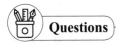 **Results and Discussions**

1. Examination of the properties of metronidazole oral ulcer film and potassium nitrate dental film. Record the inspection results in the Table 11–1.

Table 11–1　The properties of metronidazole oral ulcer film and potassium nitrate dental film

Preparations	Appearance	Thickness	Color	Bubble
Metronidazole oral ulcer film				
Potassium nitrate dental film				

2. Based on the experimental results, analyze the difference in film-forming properties between polyvinyl alcohol (17-88) and carboxymethylcellulose sodium.

Questions

1. Which film-forming methods are commonly used in the preparation of small amount of film agents? What are the key points of operation?

2. What are the role of various excipients in the formula of films?

3. How to prevent air bubbles during film preparation?

PPT

实验十二　软膏剂的制备与体外释药速率测定

实验目的

1. **掌握**　不同类型基质软膏剂的制备方法及注意事项；软膏剂释药速率的测定方法。
2. **熟悉**　不同基质对药物释放的影响。

实验原理

软膏剂系指药物与适宜基质混合制成的均匀膏状的半固体外用制剂。基质根据性质可分为油脂性、乳剂型、水溶性三类，对软膏的性状、药物释放及吸收均有重要影响。油脂性基质包括动植物油脂类、类脂类及烃类，常混合使用，以获得适宜稠度。乳剂型基质是由水相、油相借助乳化剂的乳化作用形成，根据所用乳化剂的不同，可制得 O/W 型和 W/O 型乳膏基质。水溶性基质主要由天然或合成的水溶性高分子材料所组成，常用甘油明胶、纤维素衍生物、聚乙二醇和聚丙烯酸等。软膏剂中除基质以外，还可根据具体情况，加入吸收促进剂、保湿剂、防腐剂等附加剂。

根据药物和基质的不同，软膏剂的制备可选用研和法、熔合法、乳化法。

（1）研和法　将药物粉碎后，加入少量基质或适宜液体研磨使混匀，再递加其余基质，研匀即得。适用于不耐热药物及半固体、液体成分基质的软膏剂制备。

（2）熔合法　先将基质加温熔化，再根据药物溶解性的不同，分别以固体粉末或溶液状态分次加入，边加边搅拌，直至冷却定形，即得。适用于固体药量较多或常温下不能混匀的多熔点成分基质的软膏剂制备。

（3）乳化法　先将油溶性成分加热熔化混匀，另将水溶性成分溶于水中，加热至油相相同或略高温度，两相混合乳化即得乳剂型软膏。对于在油、水两相中均不溶的药物，则需先粉碎成 100~120 目粉末，待基质形成后再分散于其中。

软膏应均匀细腻、稠度适宜，易于涂布，对皮肤和黏膜无刺激性，无酸败、变色、变硬、油水分离。释药性能是影响软膏有效性的重要指标之一。一般而言，水溶性基质和乳剂型基质中药物释放最快，烃类基质中药物释放最慢，可根据药物性质，选用不同基质以获得适宜的释药速率。软膏的释药性能可采用凝胶扩散法、离体皮肤法测定，也可通过测定药物透过无屏障性半透膜到释放介质的速度来评定。

实验器材

1. **仪器**　烧杯、研钵、水浴锅、移液管、容量瓶、试管、软膏板、软膏刀、直尺等。
2. **材料**　白凡士林、液状石蜡、硬脂醇、月桂醇硫酸钠、羟苯乙酯、甘油、蒸馏水、单硬脂酸甘油酯、聚山梨酯 80、蜂蜡、固体石蜡、司盘 80、羧甲基纤维素钠、水杨酸、水杨酸对照品、氯化钠、氯化钾、氯化钙、琼脂、三氯化铁等。

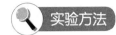 **实验方法**

（一）油脂性基质的制备

【处方】

白凡士林	10g
液状石蜡	2.5g

【制法】按处方取白凡士林与液状石蜡于软膏板上，混合均匀，即得。

【注意事项】气温变化可导致基质稠度改变，可通过适当增减液状石蜡用量以调节。

（二）乳剂型基质的制备

1. O/W 型乳剂型基质的制备

【处方】

硬脂醇	1.8g
白凡士林	2.0g
液状石蜡	1.3ml
月桂醇硫酸钠	0.2g
羟苯乙酯	0.02g
甘油	1.0g
蒸馏水	13.7ml

【制法】

（1）称取处方量油相成分（硬脂醇、白凡士林和液状石蜡）置烧杯中，水浴加热至 70~80℃ 使其熔化。

（2）称取处方量水相成分（月桂醇硫酸钠、羟苯乙酯、甘油和蒸馏水）置另一个烧杯中，水浴加热至 70~80℃。

（3）在搅拌下将水相溶液以细流状加入油相溶液中，水浴上继续保持恒温并搅拌几分钟，从水浴上取下，室温下不断搅拌至冷凝，即得。

2. W/O 型乳剂型基质的制备

【处方】

单硬脂酸甘油酯	6.0g
白凡士林	2.0g
聚山梨酯 80	0.4g
蜂蜡	2.0g
液状石蜡	10g
固体石蜡	2.0g
司盘 80	0.8g
羟苯乙酯	0.04g
蒸馏水	16.8ml

【制法】

（1）称取处方量油相成分（单硬脂酸甘油酯、白凡士林、蜂蜡、液状石蜡、固体石蜡和司盘 80）置烧杯中，水浴加热至 80℃ 使其熔化。

（2）称取处方量水相成分（聚山梨酯 80、羟苯乙酯和蒸馏水）置另一个烧杯中，水浴加热至 80℃。

（3）在搅拌下将水相溶液缓缓加入油相溶液中，水浴上恒温搅拌几分钟，再从水浴上取下，室温下不断搅拌至冷凝，即得。

【注意事项】制备过程中注意控制温度。

（三）水溶性基质的制备

【处方】

羧甲基纤维素钠	1.2g
甘油	3.0g
羟苯乙酯	0.04g
蒸馏水	15.8ml

【制法】

（1）取处方量羧甲基纤维素钠置于研钵中，加处方量甘油研磨均匀。

（2）将处方量羟苯乙酯溶于12ml蒸馏水中，再将该水溶液缓缓加入研钵，研磨均匀，加剩余蒸馏水，研磨均匀，即得。

【注意事项】羧甲基纤维素钠粉末不能直接加入水中溶解，需先用甘油研磨充分分散后再加水溶解，否则易成团而不易分散，影响基质均匀性。

（四）5%水杨酸软膏剂的制备

【处方】

水杨酸细粉	0.5g
不同类型基质	各9.5g

【制法】

（1）水杨酸油脂性软膏的制备　称取水杨酸细粉0.5g置研钵中，分次加入油脂性基质9.5g，研匀，即得。

（2）水杨酸乳膏的制备　称取水杨酸细粉0.5g置研钵中，分次加入O/W型或W/O型乳剂型基质9.5g，研匀，即得。

（3）水杨酸水溶性软膏的制备　称取水杨酸细粉0.5g置研钵中，分次加入水溶性基质9.5g，研匀，即得。

【注意事项】

（1）水杨酸需先粉碎，过100目筛。

（2）水杨酸软膏配制过程中避免接触金属器皿。

（五）软膏剂释药性能的测定

1. 林格溶液的配制

【处方】

氯化钠	1.70g
氯化钾	0.06g
氯化钙	0.066g
蒸馏水	适量

【制法】取氯化钠、氯化钾、氯化钙，溶于适量蒸馏水中，加水定容至200ml即得。

2. 含三氯化铁试液的琼脂基质配制

【处方】

琼脂	4g
林格溶液	200ml
三氯化铁试液	5ml

【制法】

（1）称取琼脂，加林格溶液200ml，沸水浴加热熔化20分钟，趁热过滤。

（2）加入三氯化铁试液（0.9→10）5ml，趁热等量分装于4支试管中，使液面距试管口约1.5cm，自然冷却后备用。

3. 不同类型软膏基质的体外释药试验

（1）取前述制得的4种水杨酸软膏，分别紧密填充于盛有琼脂基质的试管中，使软膏与基质表面紧贴而无气泡，各试管装量一致。

（2）分别于加样后1、3、5、13、16、19和24小时测量并记录试管中色区的长度L（mm）。

（3）扩散距离与时间的关系可用Lockie经验式表示：

$$L^2 = kt \tag{12-1}$$

式中，L为扩散距离（mm）；t为扩散时间（h）；k为扩散系数（mm²/h）。以不同时间色层长度的平方（L^2）对扩散时间（t）作图，可得到一条直线，直线的斜率为k，k值反映了软膏中释药速率的大小。

💬 实验结果与讨论

1. 实验结果

（1）对不同基质水杨酸软膏的均匀性、细腻度、黏稠性及涂布性进行描述。

（2）记录4种水杨酸软膏在不同时间点试管中色区的长度（表12-1），并以不同时间色层长度的平方（L^2）对扩散时间（t）分别作图，获取直线斜率k。

表 12-1　水杨酸软膏的测定结果

水杨酸软膏样品	性状	扩散距离 /mm							$k/（mm^2/h）$
		1h	3h	5h	13h	16h	19h	24h	
油脂性软膏									
O/W 型乳膏									
W/O 型乳膏									
水溶性软膏									

2. 讨论

（1）对比不同基质制备所得软膏的性状，讨论各基质对软膏均匀性、细腻度、黏稠性及涂布性的影响及其原因。

（2）对比不同基质制备所得水杨酸软膏释药曲线的k值，讨论各基质对软膏释药性能的影响及其原因。

✏️ 思考题

1. 如何进行软膏剂基质类型的选择？
2. 软膏剂制备过程中如何选择适宜的药物加入方法？
3. 乳化法制备乳剂型软膏的注意事项有哪些？
4. 影响药物从软膏基质中释放的因素有哪些？

（谢兴亮）

Lab. 12   Preparation of Ointment and Determination of Release Rate *in Vitro*

 Experimental Objectives

1. To master the preparation methods and attention points of different base types of ointments, the determination methods of release rate of ointment.

2. To be familiar with the effects of different bases on drug release.

 Experimental Principles

Ointments are semi-solid topical preparations with uniform paste shape made by mixing the drug with suitable bases. According to the properties, the bases can be divided into three types: greasy, emulsion and water-soluble, which have important effects on the characters, drug release and absorption of ointments. Greasy base includes greases and vegetable oils, lipoids, and hydrocarbons, which are often mixed to obtain a suitable consistency. Cream base is obtained by the emulsification of water phase and oil phase with the aid of emulsifiers, and O/W and W/O emulsion can be prepared according to the different emulsifiers used. The water-soluble base is mainly composed of natural or synthetic water-soluble polymer materials, and glycerol gelatin, cellulose derivatives, polyethylene glycol and polyacrylic acid are commonly used. In addition to the base, ointments can also be added in additional agents such as absorption enhancers, humectants, and preservatives according to specific conditions.

Ointments can be prepared with the grinding method or the melting method or the emulsification method according to different drugs and bases.

(1) The Grinding Method: After smashing drugs, a small amount of base or appropriate liquid is added to grind and mix well, then add the remaining base and grind evenly. This method is suitable for the preparation of ointments containing heat-labile drugs and semi-solid or liquid component bases.

(2) The Melting Method: Firstly, the base is heated to melt, and then add drugs in powder or solution state according to its solubility, while stirring, until the mixture cools down and its shape is fixed. This method is suitable for the preparation of ointments with more solid medicine or the base including multiple melting points components, which can not be evenly mixed at room temperature.

(3) The Emulsification Method: Firstly, the oil-soluble components are heated to melt and mix well, and the water-soluble components are dissolved in water, then heated to the same or slightly higher temperature of oil phase, and last the two phases are mixed and emulsified to obtain the cream. For the drugs insoluble in both oil and water, it is necessary to firstly smash them into 100~120 mesh powder, and then disperse them into the prepared base.

The ointment should be even, fine and smooth, of suitable consistency, easy to extend, not irritative to the skin and mucous membranes, and have no rancidity, discoloration, hardening, or oil-water separation. The drug release is one of the important indicators affecting the effectiveness of ointments. In general, the drug release is the fastest in the water-soluble base and cream base, and the slowest in the hydrocarbon base. Different bases can be selected to obtain the appropriate drug release rate according to the drug properties. The drug release properties of ointments can be determined by the gel diffusion method, the skin *in vitro* method or by measuring the rate of drug penetrating through the non-barrier semi-permeable film to the release medium.

 Equipments and Materials

1. Equipments   Beaker, mortar, water bath kettle, pipette, volumetric flask, test tube, ointment plate, ointment knife, ruler, etc.

2. Materials   White vaseline, liquid paraffin, stearyl alcohol, sodium lauryl sulfate, hydroxyphenethyl ester, glycerol, distilled water, glyceryl monostearate, polysorbate 80, beeswax, paraffin wax, Span 80, sodium carboxymethylcellulose, salicylic acid, salicylic acid reference substance, sodium chloride, potassium chloride, calcium chloride, agar, ferric chloride, etc.

 Experimental Methods

I. Preparation of Greasy Base

【Formula】

White vaseline	10g
Liquid paraffin	2.5g

【Procedure】According to the formula, take white vaseline and liquid paraffin on the ointment plate, mix well, then get it.

【Notes】Changes in temperature can lead to changes in base consistency, which can be adjusted by increasing or decreasing the amount of liquid paraffin.

II. Preparation of Cream Base

1. Preparation of O/W cream base

【Formula】

Stearyl alcohol	1.8g
White vaseline	2.0g
Liquid paraffin	1.3ml
Sodium lauryl sulfate	0.2g
Hydroxyphenethyl ester	0.02g
Glycerol	1.0g
Distilled water	13.7ml

【Procedure】

(1) Weigh the prescribed amount of oil phase components (stearyl alcohol, white vaseline and liquid paraffin) into a beaker, heat them to 70~80℃ in a water bath to melt them.

(2) Weigh the prescribed amount of water phase components (sodium lauryl sulfate, hydroxyphenethyl ester, glycerol, and distilled water) into another beaker and heat them to 70~80℃ in a water bath.

(3) Add the aqueous phase solution into the oily phase solution in a fine flow under stirring, keep the constant temperature in a water bath and stir for several minutes, and then remove it from the water bath, and continuously stir it to be solidified at room temperature.

2. Preparation of W/O cream base

【Formula】

Glyceryl monostearate	6.0g
White vaseline	2.0g
Polysorbate 80	0.4g
Beeswax	2.0g
Liquid paraffin	10g
Paraffin wax	2.0g
Span 80	0.8g
Hydroxyphenylethyl ester	0.04g
Distilled water	16.8ml

【Procedure】

(1) Weigh the prescribed amount of oily phase components (glyceryl monostearate, white vaseline, beeswax, liquid paraffin, paraffin wax, and Span 80) into a beaker and heat them to 80℃ in a water bath to melt them.

(2) Weigh the prescribed amount of water phase components (polysorbate 80, hydroxyphenethyl ester, and distilled water) into another beaker and heat them to 80℃ in a water bath.

(3) Add slowly the aqueous phase solution into the oily phase solution under stirring, stir at constant temperature in the water bath for a few minutes, then take it off the water bath, and continuously stir it to be solidified at room temperature.

【Notes】Pay attention to temperature control during the preparation.

III. Preparation of Water-Soluble Base

【Formula】

Sodium carboxymethylcellulose	1.2g
Glycerol	3.0g
Hydroxyphenethyl ester	0.04g
Distilled water	15.8ml

【Procedure】

(1) Place the prescribed amount of sodium carboxymethylcellulose in a mortar, add the prescribed amount of glycerol and grind evenly.

(2) Dissolve the prescribed amount of hydroxyphenethyl ester in 12ml of distilled water, and then slowly add this aqueous solution into the mortar, grind evenly, add the remaining distilled water, grind evenly, and get it.

【Notes】The powder of sodium carboxymethylcellulose can not be directly added into water for dissolution. It is necessary to use glycerol to grind and disperse it fully and then add water for dissolution. Otherwise, it is easy to form clumps and difficult to disperse, which would affect the base uniformity.

IV. Preparation of 5% Salicylic Acid Ointment

【Formula】

Salicylic acid fine powder	0.5g
Different types of bases	9.5g

【Procedure】

(1) Preparation of salicylic acid greasy ointment: 0.5g of salicylic acid fine powder was weighed and placed in a mortar, 9.5g of greasy base was added in portions, grind well, and get it.

(2) Preparation of salicylic acid emulsifiable paste: 0.5g of salicylic acid fine powder was weighed and placed in a mortar, and 9.5g of O/W or W/O cream base was added in portions, grind well, and get it.

(3) Preparation of salicylic acid water-soluble ointment: 0.5g of salicylic acid fine powder was weighed and placed in a mortar, 9.5g of water-soluble base was added in portions, in portions, grind well, and get it.

【Notes】

(1) Salicylic acid should be crushed first and passed through a 100-mesh sieve.

(2) Avoid contacting with metal ware during the preparation of salicylic acid ointments.

V. Determination of Drug Release Properties of Ointments

1. Preparation of Ringer's solution

【Formula】

Sodium chloride	1.70g
Potassium chloride	0.06g
Calcium chloride	0.066g
Distilled water	q.s.

【Procedure】Take sodium chloride, potassium chloride, and calcium chloride, dissolve them in an appropriate amount of distilled water, and add water to the constant volume of 200ml.

2. Preparation of agar base containing ferric chloride solution

【Formula】

Agar	4g
Ringer's solution	200ml
Ferric chloride solution	5ml

【Procedure】

(1) Weigh agar, add 200ml of Ringer's solution, heat and melt in boiling water bath for 20 minutes, and filter while hot.

(2) Add 5ml of ferric chloride test solution ($0.9 \rightarrow 10$), divide equally into 4 test tubes while hot, so that the liquid level is about 1.5cm away from the test tube orifice, and naturally cool them for future use.

3. *In vitro* drug release test of different types of ointment bases

(1) Take the four kinds of salicylic acid ointments prepared above, and fill them tightly in test tubes containing agar base respectively, so that the ointments and the surface of the base are close without bubbles, and the filling amount of each test tube is the same.

(2) Measure and record the length (L, mm) of the color zone in the test tube at 1, 3, 5, 13, 16, 19 and 24 hours after sample addition.

(3) The relationship between diffusion distance and time can be expressed by the Lockie empirical formula:

$$L^2=kt \tag{12-1}$$

In formula: L is the diffusion distance (mm), t is the diffusion time (h), k is the diffusion coefficient (mm^2/h). A straight line can be obtained by plotting the diffusion time (t) with the square (L^2) of the length of the color layer at different times, the slope of the straight line is k, and the value of k reflects the drug release rate of ointments.

Results and Discussions

1. Results

(1) Describe the uniformity, fineness, viscosity and coating of salicylic acid ointment with different bases.

(2) Record the length of the color zone in the test tube at different time points for the four kinds of salicylic acid ointments (Table 12–1), and plot the diffusion time (t) with the square (L^2) of the length of the color layer at different times, respectively, to obtain the slope k.

Table 12–1　Determination results of salicylic acid ointments

Samples of Salicylic Acid Ointments	Appearance	Diffusion distance/mm							$k/(mm^2/h)$
		1h	3h	5h	13h	16h	19h	24h	
Greasy ointment									
O/W cream									
W/O cream									
Water-soluble ointment									

2. Discussions

(1) Compare the properties of ointments prepared with different bases, and discuss the effects of each base on the uniformity, fineness, viscosity and spreadability of ointments and their reasons.

(2) Compare the k values of the release curves of salicylic acid ointments prepared from different bases, and discuss the effect of each base on the release properties of ointments and its causes.

 Questions

1. How to select the base of ointments?
2. How to select the suitable drug addition method during ointment preparation?
3. What are the attention points for the preparation of cream?
4. What are the factors that affect the drug release from the ointment base?

实验十三　中药制剂的制备

PPT

实验目的

1. **掌握**　中药制剂及其常用剂型的特点；中药常见剂型的制备方法。
2. **熟悉**　常用中药浸提方法及适用范围。
3. **了解**　影响中药制剂质量的因素。

实验原理

中药制剂是指在中医药理论指导下，按照中药性质、用药目的及给药途径，依据《中国药典》等的规定，将中药原料经加工后制成的具有一定规格标准，可以直接用于防病治病的药品。由于通常采用中药饮片作为原料，中药制剂生产过程需要首先对原料进行粉碎、过筛、混合以及浸提、精制、浓缩等处理，方能进一步加工制成不同剂型的产品。因此，中药有其独特的剂型，如各种浸出制剂、丸剂、胶剂、颗粒剂等。中药制剂的质量不仅取决于中药原料自身的品质，且受到上述处理过程的直接影响。

中药浸出制剂是指采用适当的溶剂和方法，从中药饮片中浸出有效成分，经适当精制与浓缩得到的供内服或外用的一类制剂。包括汤剂、合剂、口服液、糖浆剂、煎膏剂、酒剂、酊剂、流浸膏剂与浸膏剂等。

中药合剂是指药材用水或其他溶剂，采用适宜方法提取、纯化、浓缩制成的内服液体制剂（单剂量灌装者称"口服液"）。中药合剂的制备工艺流程为：浸出→净化→浓缩→分装→灭菌等。

煎膏剂系是指药材用水煎煮，取煎煮液浓缩，加炼蜜或糖（或转化糖）制成的半流体制剂，所加炼蜜或糖的量，一般不超过清膏量的3倍。

流浸膏剂系指药材用适宜的溶剂提取，蒸去部分溶剂，调整浓度至规定标准而制成的制剂。除另有规定外，流浸膏剂每1ml相当于原药材1g。流浸膏剂直接作为制剂服用较少，一般多用作配制酊剂、合剂、糖浆剂、丸剂及其他制剂的原料。流浸膏剂除特殊规定外，一般都以不同浓度乙醇为溶剂，用渗漉法制备，有时也用浸渍法和煎煮法制备，亦可用浸膏剂加规定溶剂稀释制成。

丸剂是指药材细粉或提取物加适宜的黏合剂或其他辅料制成的（类）球形固体制剂。其制备方法包括泛制法、塑制法和滴制法。中药丸剂包括蜜丸、水丸、水蜜丸、糊丸、蜡丸、浓缩丸、滴丸等。其中蜜丸是将药材细粉以炼制过的蜂蜜为黏合剂制成的丸剂，常用塑制法。炼蜜的目的在于除去杂质，破坏酶类，杀死微生物，减少水分，增加黏合力。根据炼制程度可将炼蜜分为嫩蜜、中蜜和老蜜，制备蜜丸时应根据药料性质、气候温度等选用适宜的炼蜜类型和用量，使所得蜜丸细腻滋润、软硬适中。

颗粒剂系指药物或药材提取物与适宜的辅料或药材细粉制成的干燥颗粒状固体制剂。一般制备工艺流程为：原辅料的处理→制软材→制颗粒→干燥→整粒→质量检查→包装。

⚙ **实验器材**

1. **仪器** 天平、渗漉筒、挥发油提取器、漏斗、烧杯、量筒、电炉、药筛、玻璃棒等。
2. **材料** 益母草、远志、黄芪、防风、白术（炒）、山楂、麦芽（炒）、六神曲（麸炒）、板蓝根、乙醇、红糖、蔗糖、蜂蜜、糖粉、糊精、蒸馏水、滤纸、脱脂棉等。

🔍 **实验方法**

（一）益母草膏的制备
【处方】

益母草	200g
红糖	50g

【制法】

（1）取益母草，切碎，加水煎煮两次，每次2小时，滤过，合并滤液，滤液浓缩至相对密度为1.21~1.25（80℃）的清膏。

（2）称取红糖，加入糖量1/2的水，加热熬炼，不断搅拌，至糖成深红色时，停止加热，将清膏缓慢加入其中，搅拌混匀，继续用文火加热浓缩至规定的相对密度，即得。

【性状】本品为棕黑色稠厚的半流体；气微，味苦、甜。

【功能与主治】活血调经。用于血瘀所致的月经不调、产后恶露不绝，症见月经量少、淋漓不尽、产后出血时间过长；产后子宫复旧不全见上述证候者。

【注意事项】

（1）益母草提取时间长，故浓缩时，应不断搅拌，注意防止糊化。

（2）本品的相对密度应不低于1.36。

（二）远志流浸膏的制备
【处方】

远志	100g
60%乙醇	适量成100ml

【制法】取远志粗粉，用60%乙醇作溶剂，按渗漉法制备，浸渍24小时后，以每分钟1~3ml的速度缓缓渗漉，收集初漉液85ml，另器保存，继续渗漉至有效成分完全漉出，收集续漉液，在60℃以下浓缩至稠膏状，加入初滤液，混匀，滴加浓氨试液适量使显微碱性（pH约为8），并有氨臭，用60%乙醇调整浓度至每1ml相当于原药材1g，静置，待澄清后滤过，即得。

【性状】本品为棕色的液体，振摇后产生泡沫。

【用途】远志酊的原料。

【注意事项】

（1）远志含三萜酸性皂苷——远志皂苷，水解后生成远志皂苷元及糖。为避免远志酸性皂苷的水解，在渗漉过程中需加入氨溶液，防止皂苷元沉淀析出。

（2）装筒前，应先用溶剂将药粉充分润湿。装筒时应分次投入，逐层压平，做到松紧均匀。投料完毕用滤纸或纱布覆盖，加少许干净碎石以防止药材松动。筒中空气应尽量排除干净。

（3）本品含醇量应为38%~48%。

（三）玉屏风口服液的制备
【处方】

黄芪	60g

| 防风 | 20g |
| 白术（炒） | 20g |

【制法】

（1）将防风碎断，提取挥发油，蒸馏后的药液另器收集，备用。

（2）药渣与黄芪、白术混合，加水煎煮两次，第一次1.5小时，第二次1小时，合并煎液，滤过。

（3）滤液浓缩至适量（约100ml），加乙醇使含醇量为60%，静置，滤过，滤液回收乙醇，加水搅匀，静置，取上清液滤过，滤液浓缩（约20ml）。

（4）取蔗糖40g制成糖浆（约50ml），与上述浓缩液合并，再加入挥发油及蒸馏后的药液，调节总量至100ml，混匀，滤过，灌封（每支10ml），灭菌，即得。

【性状】本品为棕红色至棕褐色的液体；味甜、微苦、涩。

【功能与主治】益气，固表，止汗。用于表虚不固，自汗恶风，面色㿠白或体虚易感风邪者。

【注意事项】本品相对密度应不低于1.16。pH应为4.0~5.5。

（四）大山楂丸的制备

【处方】

山楂	100g
麦芽（炒）	15g
六神曲（麸炒）	15g

【制法】

（1）以上3味，粉碎成细粉，过7号筛，混匀。

（2）称取蔗糖60g，加水27ml煮沸使溶解，加入蜂蜜60g混合，炼至比重约为1.38（70℃）、手捻有一定黏性而无长丝，趁热以脱脂棉过滤。

（3）取适量炼蜜与上述粉末混合（每100g药粉用蜜量约为90g），揉搓制成均匀滋润的丸块；根据搓丸板规格将药坨分块并搓成适宜丸条，再用搓丸板搓圆成丸。

【性状】本品为棕红色至褐色的大蜜丸；味酸、甜。

【功能与主治】开胃消食。用于食积内停所致的食欲不振、消化不良、脘腹胀闷等症。

【注意事项】

（1）炼蜜时应注意炼制程度，根据药物性质控制加热时间、温度、颜色、水分等；炼制过程中应不断搅拌，避免溢出；并趁热过滤。

（2）和药时应采用温蜜，并使药粉与炼蜜充分混匀，制成软硬适度、可塑性佳的丸块，以利进一步搓丸条、制丸块。

（3）预先在搓条、搓丸工具上涂抹适量润滑剂，可以避免粘连，确保丸粒表面光滑。可用麻油100g加入蜂蜡20~30g熔融制成润滑剂。

（五）板蓝根颗粒的制备

【处方】

板蓝根	50g
糖粉	30g
糊精	10g
乙醇	适量

【制法】

（1）取板蓝根加水适量浸泡1小时，煎煮2次（2小时、1小时），合并煎液，滤过。

（2）滤液浓缩至约50ml，加乙醇使含醇量达60%，搅匀，静置过夜。

（3）取上清液回收乙醇，并浓缩至相对密度为1.30~1.33（80℃）的清膏（约35g）。

91

（4）取糖粉和糊精过80目筛混匀，逐渐加入清膏中制成软材，过14目筛制颗粒，60℃干燥，过10目筛整粒，即得。

【性状】本品为黄棕色颗粒；味甜、微苦。

【功能与主治】清热解毒、凉血利咽。用于肺胃热盛所致的咽喉肿痛、口咽干燥、腮部肿胀；急性扁桃体炎、腮腺炎见上述证候者等。

【注意事项】制软材时应软硬适宜，"手握成团、轻压即散"，可加入少量乙醇调节。

实验结果与讨论

1. 请将上述浸出制剂的性状检查结果填入表 13-1。

表 13-1　益母草膏、远志流浸膏及玉屏风口服液性状检查结果

制剂	颜色	嗅味	pH	相对密度
益母草膏				
远志流浸膏				
玉屏风口服液				

2. 记录所得大山楂丸的外观性状，并检查其重量差异。

3. 记录所得板蓝根颗粒的外观性状，并检查其溶化性（取 10g 颗粒，加热水 200ml，搅拌 5 分钟，应全部溶化，允许有轻微浑浊）。

4. 试分析玉屏风口服液处方中防风提取挥发油、黄芪及白术水煎煮提取的依据。提取液醇沉的目的是什么？

思考题

1. 比较浸渍、渗漉、回流等中药提取方法的优缺点，讨论各法的适应范围以及操作关键。

2. 煎膏剂制备过程中应注意哪些问题？如何防止煎膏剂的"返砂"？

3. 浸提药剂中哪些剂型需测定含醇量？测定含醇量有何意义？

4. 中药颗粒剂制备过程中应注意哪些问题？

5. 中药制剂与现代药物制剂有何异同点？请查阅相关资料、深入思考并与同学讨论。

（王文苹）

Lab. 13 Pharmaceutical Preparations of Chinese Materia Medica

 Experimental Objectives

1. To master the features for pharmaceutical preparations of Chinese Materia Medica and their commonly-used dosage forms.

2. To be familiar with the common extraction methods for Chinese Materia Medica and their application.

3. To understand the key factors influencing preparation quality of Chinese Materia Medica.

 Experimental Principles

Preparations of Chinese Materia Medica are pharmaceutical products with certain specification developed under the guidance of Chinese medicinal theory, and they can be directly applied for precautionary or therapeutic purposes. These preparations are processed from Chinese crude drugs in accordance with the regulation of *Chinese Pharmacopoeia* and the property of crude drugs, medication goals and administration routes. Since medicinal slices of Chinese crude drugs are generally served as the raw material, it must be pretreated before further processed to be pharmaceutical products in different dosage forms. The pretreating procedure includes grinding, sieving, mixing, extraction, purification and concentration. Therefore, Chinese medicine has its unique dosage forms, including extractive preparations, pills, gelatin and granules, etc. The preparation quality of Chinese Materia Medica is depended on not only the quality of crude drug itself, but also the above-mentioned treating processes.

Extractive preparations of Chinese Medicine are a series of preparations for oral or topical application, which contains active ingredients extracted from medicinal slices of Chinese Crude Drugs with suitable solvents and by appropriate methods, followed by proper purification and concentrating process. These preparations include decoctions, mixtures, oral liquids, syrups, concentrated decoctions, medicinal wines, tinctures, fluidextracts and extracts, etc.

Mixtures of Chinese Medicine are liquid preparations for oral administration prepared by extraction with water or other solvents, purification and concentration processes. Mixtures packaged at a single dose are called as "oral liquids". Their general preparation process is described as follows: Extraction → purification → concentration → sub-packaging → sterilization.

Concentrated decoctions is a kind of semi-fluid preparations which prepared by decocting medicinal slices with water followed by concentration and addition of processed honey or sugar (or inverted sugar). The amount of processed honey or sugar is usually no more than 3 times of that of the related extract.

Fluidextracts are preparations at specified content, which produced by extracting drug with suitable solvent and evaporating part of the solvent. Unless otherwise specified, 1ml of fluidextract is equivalent

93

to 1g crude drug. Fluidextracts are seldom administrated as preparations, but more frequently applied as the raw materials for production of tinctures, mixtures, syrups, pills and other dosage forms. Unless otherwise specified, fluidextracts were prepared by percolation method (sometimes by maceration or decoction method) with ethanol at different concentrations, or by diluting extracts with required solvents.

Pills are solid preparations in (almost) spherical shapes, which made of crude drug powders or extracts with suitable binders or other excipients. Pills of Chinese Medicine include honeyed pills, watered pills, water-honeyed pills, starched pills, wax pills, concentrated pills and dripping pills, etc. Honeyed pills are made of fine powder of crude drugs with processed honey as the binder, usually prepared by rubbing method. The processing of honey before use aims to remove impurities, destroy enzymes, kill microbes, lower water content and increase adhesive strength. Depending on the degree of processing, the processed honey can be categorized into primary, secondary and tertiary processed honey. For production of honey pills in fine and smooth appearance and with moderate softness-hardness, suitable type and amount of processed honey must be selected according to the property of crude drugs and climatic temperature.

Granules are solid preparations made of drugs or extracts and suitable excipients in dry granular forms of certain size. Their general preparation process is listed as follows: Treatment of drugs and excipients → making soft materials → preparation of wet granules → drying → sieving → quality inspection → packaging.

 Equipments and Materials

1. Equipments　Balance, percolator, volatile oil extractor, funnel, beaker, measuring cylinder, induction cooker, sieve, glass rod, etc.

2. Materials　Leonuri Herba, Polygalae Radix, Astragali Radix, Saposhnikoviae Radix, Macrocephalae Rhizoma (fried), Cretaegi Fructus, Hordei Fructus Germinatus (fried), Liushenqu (fried with bran), Indigowoad Root, ethanol, brown sugar, sucrose, honey, powdered sugar, dextrin, distilled water, filter paper, degreasing cotton, etc.

 Experimental Methods

I. Preparation of Motherwort Herb Concentrated Decoction

【Formula】

| Leonuri Herba | 200g |
| Brown sugar | 50g |

【Procedure】

(1) Cut Leonuri Herba into pieces and place into the beaker. Add water and decoct the crude drug for 2 times, 2h each time. Filter and combine the decoctions. Concentrate the decoction to be a thin extract with a relative density of 1.21~1.25 at 80℃.

(2) Weigh the brown sugar and add water (1/2 amount of sugar). Melt and cook by direct heating under continuous stirring until its color turns into deep red. Add the above extract, fully mix them by stirring, and continuously concentrate over a gentle heat to the specified relative density.

【Description】A brownish-black and thick semifluid with slight odor, tastes bitter and sweet.

【 Actions and Indications 】 To active blood and regulate menstruation. Commonly used for menstrual irregularities and postpartum persistent flow of the lochia due to blood stasis, manifested as scanty menstruation, extended cycles, or prolonged postpartum hemorrhage. Postpartum subinvolution of uterus with the symptoms described above.

【 Notes 】

(1) The extract and its mixture with sugar need to be continuously stirred during the long-term heating process to avoid burning.

(2) The relative density for the final product should be no less than 1.36.

II. Preparation of Polygala Liquid Extract

【 Formula 】

Polygalae Radix	100g
60% ethanol	q.s. to 100ml

【 Procedure 】 Extract the Polygalae Radix (coarse powder) using 60% ethanol as the solvent by percolation method. Macerate for 24h, and then percolate slowly at a speed of 1~3ml/min to collect 85ml of the initial percolate. Continue the percolation until the active components are completely extracted. Collect the subsequent percolate into another container and concentrate into a thick extract by heating at below 60℃. Then mix the concentrate with the initial percolate, add dropwise a proper amount of concentrated ammonia test solution to make the mixture slightly alkaline (pH≈8) with an ammonia odor. Adjust with 60% ethanol to a required concentration of 1g crude drug per 1ml. Allow to stand until a clear supernatant is observed, and then filter to get the final product.

【 Description 】 A brown liquid with foams after shaking.

【 Application 】 Raw material for polygala tincture.

【 Notes 】

(1) The polygalacin, an acid triterpenoidsaponin in Polygalae Radix can be hydrolyzed to be tenuigenin and sugars. Therefore, ammonia must be added during the process to avoid the hydrolyzation of saponin and precipitation of sapogenin.

(2) The crude drug need to be fully moistened by the extracting solvent, then be gradually filled into the percolator and pressed layer by layer. To avoid movement of the crude drugs during the percolation process, one piece of filer paper or gauze along with some clean pebbles can be used to cover the materials. Besides, the air in percolator should be eliminated as completely as possible.

(3) The ethanol content of the obtained product should be in a range of 38%~48%.

III. Preparation of Yupingfeng Mixture

【 Formula 】

Astragali Radix	60g
Saposhnikoviae Radix	20g
Macrocephalae Rhizoma (fried)	20g

【 Procedure 】

(1) Crush the Saposhnikoviae Radix to a proper size, extract its volatile oil using the distillation method and collect the obtained distillate in a container.

(2) Mix the residue of Saposhnikoviae Radix with Astragali Radix and Macrocephalae Rhizoma (fried) and add a proper amount of water. Decoct the crude drugs twice for 1.5h and 1h respectively.

(3) Filter and combine the decoction, and concentrate to be approximately 100ml. Add ethanol until the ethanol content reaches up to 60%, and then stand until a clear supernatant is observed. Filter and

collect the filtrate, then recover the ethanol. Add water and stir the mixture, and stand for a while. Collect the supernatant and concentrate to be around 20ml.

(4) Take 40g sucrose and process it to be syrup (approximately 50ml). Mix the syrup and the above concentrated extract, then add the volatile oil and decoction after distillation. After mix well and adjust the total volume to be 100ml, filter, fill and sealing (10ml each), sterilization to obtain the final product.

【Description】A brown-red to dark brown liquid; tastes sweet, slightly bitter and puckery.

【Actions and Indications】To tonify qi, secure the exterior, and check sweating. Commonly used for pattern of exterior insecurity and qi deficiency, manifested as spontaneous sweating, aversion to wind, and bright pale complexion. Patient of weak constitution susceptible to wind pathogen.

【Notes】The final product should be with a relative density of no less than 1.16 and a pH value in a range of 4.0~5.5.

IV. Preparation of Dashanzha Pills

【Formula】

Cretaegi Fructus	100g
Hordei Fructus Germinatus (fried)	15g
Liushenqu (fried with bran)	15g

【Procedure】

(1) Crush the raw materials into fine powder over a 120-mesh sieve, and then fully mix them all.

(2) Dissolve 60g sucrose in 27ml water by boiling. Then add 60g honey and concentrate to be a sticky liquid (but no long filament between fingers) with a relative density of 1.38 at 70℃. Filter the hot mixture through degreased cotton.

(3) Mix the above powder and the processed honey at a weight ratio of 100:90 to make a pill mass with uniform and lenitive appearance. Split the pill mass and make stripes with suitable size, and then roll the stripes into pellets on the rubbing plate.

【Description】Big honeyed pills with a brownish-red to brown color, tastes sour and sweet.

【Actions and Indications】To boost appetite and promote digestion. Commonly used for poor appetite, indigestion, distension and fullness in the epigastrium and abdomen due to internal food retention.

【Notes】

(1) The heating duration, temperature, color and water content of honey must be carefully controlled to obtain the desirable degree of processing and meet the requirement of the properties of crude drugs.

(2) The warm or hot processed honey is needed to make a pill mass with suitable hardness and plasticity, which is beneficial for further preparation of pill stripes and pellets.

(3) A small amount of lubricant can be previously applied on the Equipments for stripes and pellets to avoid adhesion and to assure a smooth surface of the final pills. The lubricant can be obtained by mixing and melting 20~30g beewax with 100g sesame oil.

V. Preparation of Banlangen Granules

【Formula】

Indigowoad Root	50g
Powdered sugar	30g
Dextrin	10g
Ethanol	q.s.

【Procedure】

(1) Soak Indigowoad Root in water for 1h, then decoct it for twice (2h and 1h), and collect the decoction by filtration.

(2) Heat and concentrate the decoction to around 50ml, add ethanol to reach an ethanol content of 60%. Stir the mixture and then let it standing overnight.

(3) Collect the supernatant to recycle the ethanol, and then concentrate to be a thin extract (about 35g) with its relative density in the range of 1.30~1.33 (80℃).

(4) Mix the powdered sugar and dextrin by a 80-mesh sieve. Gradually add the powder into the thin extract and make it into a wet mass. Pass the mass through a 14-mesh sieve to obtain the granules followed by drying at 60℃. Pass the granules through a 10-mesh sieve to get the final product.

【Description】Yellowish-brown granules, tastes sweet and light bitter.

【Actions and Indications】To Clear heat, remove toxin, cool the blood aspect and soothe the throat. Commonly used for swollen sore throat, dryness in mouth and throat, and swollen cheeks due to exuberant heat of lung and stomach. Acute tonsillitis and paratotis with the symptoms described above.

【Notes】The wet mass should be with moderate softness and hardness, and can be "lumped by griping in hand, scattered by slight press". A small amount of ethanol can be added during the process.

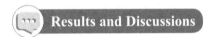 **Results and Discussions**

1. Fill the quality inspection results of the obtained preparations in the Table 13-1.

Table 13-1　Results of quality inspection for the obtained extractive preparations

Preparation	Color	Odor	pH	Relative density
Motherwort Herb Concentrated Decoction				
Polygala Liquid Extract				
Yupingfeng Mixture				

2. Record the appearance of the obtained Dashanzha Pills and examine their weight variation.

3. Record the appearance of the obtained Banlangen Granules and examine their dissolubility (take 10g granules and add 200ml hot water, then stir for 5min, it should be fully dissolved, a slight turbid is allowed).

4. Try to analyze the reasons for volatile oil extraction of Saposhnikoviae Radix, decoction of Astragali Radix and Macrocephalae Rhizoma (fried) in the formula of Yupingfeng Mixture. And discuss the purposes of ethanol precipitation of the obtained decoction.

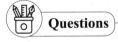 **Questions**

1. Compare the advantages and disadvantages of pickling, percolation and refluxing methods for extraction of Chinese Materia Medica. And describe the application scope and key operating steps for these methods.

2. What are the precautions during the preparation of concentrated decoctions? How to prevent the re-crystallization/sand-returning phenomenon？

3. Which dosage forms of extractive preparations are required for test of ethanol content? What is the significance for ethanol content test?

4. What are the precautions during the preparation of granules of Chinese Materia Medica?

5. What are the similarities and differences between preparations of Chinese Materia Medica and modern pharmaceutical preparations. Please discuss the question with your classmates after reading the related materials and deep thinking by yourself.

实验十四　固体分散体的制备及验证

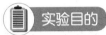 **实验目的**

1. **掌握**　熔融法制备固体分散体的工艺。
2. **熟悉**　固体分散体的鉴定方法。

实验原理

固体分散体（solid dispersion，SD）是将分子型、无定形或微晶状态的药物高度分散在适宜的载体材料中所形成的固体分散体系。按照制备方法和药物的分散状态分为低共熔混合物、固体溶液和共沉淀物等。采用水溶性载体材料则可以实现减小药物粒径、增加表面积、提高药物的分散度、增加药物的溶出速度的目的；如使用难溶性或肠溶性高分子辅料则可以利用载体限制溶出达到缓释或肠溶的目的，固体分散体的作用因此得以进一步拓展。固体分散体作为固体制剂的一种中间体，可添加适当辅料后，再经过适宜的制备工艺制成颗粒剂、胶囊剂、片剂等剂型。

常用的固体分散体材料有如下几种。①水溶性载体材料：通常为高分子聚合物、表面活性剂、有机酸及糖等，其中较为常用的有聚乙烯吡咯烷酮（PVP）、聚乙二醇类（PEG）等。②难溶性载体材料：常用的有乙基纤维素、聚丙烯酸酯类、脂质类。③肠溶性载体材料：常用的有纤维素类、聚丙烯酸树酯、脂类。

固体分散体的制备方法具体如下。

（1）熔融法是将药物与载体材料混匀，加热至熔融，将熔融物在剧烈搅拌下迅速冷却至固体，或将熔融物倒在预冷的不锈钢板上，使成薄层，在板的另一面吹冷空气或用冰使骤冷迅速成固体，然后将混合物固体在一定温度下放置，使变脆易于粉碎。

（2）溶剂法系将药物与载体材料共同溶于有机溶剂中，蒸去有机溶剂后使药物与载体材料同时析出，得到共沉淀固体分散体，经干燥即得。

（3）溶剂–熔融法是将药物溶于少量有机溶剂中，然后将此溶液加入已熔融的载体中搅拌均匀，蒸去有机溶剂，冷却固化后得到固体分散体。药物溶液在固体分散体中所占的量一般不超过10%（g/g），否则难以形成脆而易碎的固体。

固体分散体的形成可以通过测定药物溶解度和溶出速度的变化、热分析法、X射线衍射法、红外分光光度法、扫描电镜观察法、核磁共振波谱法等来分析鉴定。

实验器材

1. **仪器**　电子天平、紫外–可见分光光度计等。
2. **材料**　坩埚、研钵、微孔滤膜、量瓶、PEG 6000、布洛芬、NaOH、蒸馏水等。

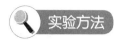 **实验方法**

（一）布洛芬固体分散体的制备

【处方】

布洛芬	0.5g
PEG 6000	4.5g

【制法】

（1）熔融法制备固体分散体　按处方量称取布洛芬及 PEG 6000，于坩埚中混匀，置电炉上加热至熔融；将熔融物倒在不锈钢盘上（盘下放置冰块），使成薄层，熔融物骤冷迅速成固体，冷却 10 分钟，粉碎，即得。

（2）物理混合物的制备　按处方量称取布洛芬及 PEG 6000，于乳钵中研磨混合均匀，即得。

【注意事项】

（1）为防止湿气的引入，加热应避免采用水浴锅加热。加热温度控制在辅料熔点以上，但温度不宜过高，时间也不宜过长，以免对药物和辅料的稳定性造成影响。

（2）熔融法制备固体分散体的关键在于熔融物料的骤冷，故将熔融的物料倾倒在不锈钢盘内，不锈钢盘置于冰上。为保持冷却过程中的干燥环境，将此盘置于冰箱冷冻室内保存。粉碎和称量操作注意快速进行，以免吸潮。

（二）布洛芬溶解度的测定

1. **标准曲线的制备**　精密称取布洛芬对照品 30mg 于 50ml 量瓶中，用 0.4% NaOH 溶液溶解并稀释至刻度，摇匀。精密吸取上述溶液 1.0、3.0、5.0、7.0、9.0ml 于 10ml 量瓶中，用 0.4% NaOH 溶液稀释至刻度，摇匀。于 265nm 处测定吸光度（A）。求出标准曲线回归方程，备用。

2. **布洛芬原料药溶解度的测定**　精密称取 0.05g 布洛芬的原料药，加水 20ml，搅拌 5 分钟，以 0.45μm 微孔滤膜过滤，取续滤液 9ml 于 10ml 的容量瓶中，加 4% 的 NaOH 溶液稀释至刻度，摇匀。在波长为 265nm 处测定吸光度，记为 A_1。

3. **物理混合物中布洛芬溶解度的测定**　精密称取 0.5g 布洛芬的物理混合物（相当于 0.05g 布洛芬），加水 20ml，搅拌 5 分钟，以 0.45μm 微孔滤膜过滤，取续滤液 9ml 于 10ml 的容量瓶中，加 4% 的 NaOH 溶液稀释至刻度，摇匀。在波长为 265nm 处测定吸光度，记为 A_2。

4. **固体分散体中布洛芬溶解度的测定**　精密称取 0.5g 布洛芬的固体分散体（相当于 0.05g 布洛芬），加水 20ml，搅拌 5 分钟，以 0.45μm 微孔滤膜过滤，取续滤液 9ml 于 10ml 的容量瓶中，加 4% 的 NaOH 溶液稀释至刻度，摇匀。在波长为 265nm 处测定吸光度，记为 A_3。

将以上三种物料的吸光度带入标准曲线回归方程，计算每种样品布洛芬的溶解度。

5. **DSC 法扫描固体分散体吸热曲线**　各取约为 5.0mg 的布洛芬 PEG 6000 固体分散体、布洛芬与 PEG 6000 的物理混合物（同固体分散体中比例）、布洛芬以及 PEG 6000，置于坩埚内。DSC 条件具体如下：以 $\alpha\text{-}Al_2O_3$ 为参比物，升温速率为 10℃/min，升温范围：25~350℃，氮气保护。通过图谱吸热曲线变化观察各种样品，特别是布洛芬固体分散体与布洛芬与 PEG 6000 的物理混合物的差异。

【注意事项】 溶解度的测定中，时间均为搅拌 5 分钟平行操作，以 5 分钟的溶出量来测定布洛芬原料药、物理混合物、固体分散体中布洛芬的溶解度。

实验结果与讨论

1. **结果**

（1）布洛芬原料药、物理混合物、固体分散体中布洛芬溶解度的测定结果见表 14-1 所示。

表 14-1　布洛芬原料药、物理混合物、固体分散体中布洛芬溶解度的测定结果

样品	A 值	溶解度
原料药		
物理混合物		
固体分散体		

（2）绘制布洛芬原料药、物理混合物、固体分散体中布洛芬 DSC 曲线。

2. 讨论

（1）比较三个样品的溶解度，并对此做出合理解释。

（2）本实验中测定溶解度时，每种样品溶出均为搅拌 5 分钟，时间上如此控制有何意义？

思考题

1. PEG 6000 在使用时是否需要粉碎过筛？其粒径大小对物理混合物及固体分散体中布洛芬的溶解度是否有影响？

2. 简述固体分散体速释和缓释的原理。

3. 固体分散体在贮藏期内容易发生老化现象，采用什么方法可以延缓其老化，提高其稳定性？

（彭海生）

Lab. 14 — Preparation and Evaluation of Solid Dispersion

Experimental Objectives

1. To master the preparation process of solid dispersion formulation by melting method.
2. To be familiar with the identification methods of solid dispersion products.

Experimental Principles

Solid dispersion (SD) is a molecular, amorphous, or microcrystalline dispersion of an active ingredients evenly dispersed in a solid matrix of suitable carrier including water soluble or poorly soluble materials. According to the preparation method and the dispersion status of drug, the preparation methods are classified as followed: eutectic mixture, solid solution, and coprecipitates. The water soluble carriers can reduce the size of water poorly soluble ingredients, increase the specific area of particle, and improve the degree of dispersion of SD, resulting in the increased dissolution of hydrophobic drug. On the contrary, water poorly soluble carrier or enteric soluble polymers can decrease the dissolution of hydrophilic drug to achieve the aim of sustained or enteric liquid-triggered release. The application of SD technique has been widened and deepened accordingly. SD could be also used as an intermediate to prepare the granules, capsules, and tables, etc, when mixes with suitable additives followed the reasonable preparation process.

The commonly-used carriers are as followed: ①water soluble additives: polymers, surfactants, organic acid, etc, of which the most commonly-used materials are polyvinylpyrrolidone (PVP), polyethylene glycol (PEG), etc; ②water poorly soluble additives: ethyl cellulose, polyacrylic acid esters, and lipids are the commonly-used materials; ③ enteric carriers: cellulose and polyacrylic acid esters with enteric capability are the commonly-used materials.

The preparation methods of SD are as under:

(1) Melting Method: Mix active ingredients with additives evenly, heat to fusion, stir vigorously to cooling down to solid status, or pour the melt mixtures on a pre-cooling stainless steel plate, make them a thin layer and then blow from the opposite side of the plate with cold air or cooling down the opposite side of plate with ice bath to make the mixtures rapidly solidification. Finally, put the mixtures aside at a given temperature, make them fragile and easy to crush.

(2) Solvent Method: Put ingredients and additives into a given solvent and make them dissolved, evaporate the solvent and precipitate, obtain the co-precipitation SD and then dry them for use.

(3) Solvent-Helting Method: Put active ingredients into small amount of organic solvent, add the solution into the melt carrier liquid, stir evenly and evaporate the solvent, then cooling down the mixture to obtain the SD. Generally, the ratio of solution containing drug to the SD is less 10% (g/g). Otherwise, it is difficult to form the fragile and easy-to-crush solid.

Identification of CD can be performed by the methods such as measuring solubility or dissolution of a drug, thermal analysis, X-ray diffraction, infrared spectrophotometry, scanning electron microscopy, and nuclear magnetic resonance spectroscopy, etc.

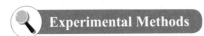

Equipments and Materials

1. Equipments Electronic balance, ultraviolet spectrophotometer, etc.

2. Materials Crucible, mortar, microporous filter membrane, volumetric flask, PEG 6000, ibuprofen, NaOH, distilled water, etc.

Experimental Methods

I. Preparation of Ibuprofen CD

【Formula】

Ibuprofen	0.5g
PEG 6000	4.5g

【Procedure】

(1) Melting method to prepare ibuprofen SD: Weigh ibuprofen and PEG 6000 according to the formula and put them into a crucible, mix evenly, and put crucible on an electric stove and heat to melt. Pour the melted mixture on a stainless steel tray incubated with ice, and make it a thin layer, then the melted materials rapidly solidify for 10 mins, crush the solid to obtain ibuprofen SD.

(2) Preparation method of physical mixture, weigh ibuprofen and PEG 6000 according to the formula and put them into a mortar, mix evenly, obtain physical mixture.

【Notes】

(1) To avoid absorption of moisture, water bath should not be used. To avoid the influence of active ingredients and additives, heating temperature should be slightly higher than melting points of additives to dissolve ibuprofen but the temperature should be controlled at a reasonable range and heating time should be not too long.

(2) The key steps of melting method for ibuprofen SD is shock cooling. Hence the melted materials should be poured the pre-cooling stainless steel tray on the ice. To keep the dry environment around materials, the tray should be put at a freezer room of refrigerator before use. To avoid absorption of moisture, quick operation of crushing and weighing should be performed.

II. Measurement of Ibuprofen Solubility

1. Standard curve Precisely weigh 30mg of standard product of ibuprofen and put it into 50ml of volumetric flask, dissolve it with 0.4% NaOH solution, dilute to 50ml and shake well. Accurately pipette the above-mentioned solution of 1.0, 3.0, 5.0, 7.0 and 9.0ml and transfer to 10ml of volumetric flask, dilute the solution with 0.4% NaOH to 10ml, shake well. Detect the absorbance of solution at 265nm (A), draw standard curve and calculate regression equation for use.

2. Measurement of the solubility of raw ibuprofen Precisely weigh 0.05g of raw ibuprofen, add 20ml of water, keep stirring for 5 mins and then filter the solution with microporous filter (0.45μm). Pipette 9ml of continuous filtrate and transfer to 10ml of volumetric flask, add 4% NaOH solution to 10ml, shake well. Detect the absorbance of solution at 265nm (A_1).

3. Measurement of the solubility of physical mixture   Precisely weigh 0.5g of physical mixture of ibuprofen and PEG 6000 (calculated as ibuprofen, 0.05g), add 20ml of water, keep stirring for 5 mins and then filter the solution with microporous filter (0.45μm). Pipette 9ml of continuous filtrate and transfer to 10ml of volumetric flask, add 4% NaOH solution to 10ml, shake well. Detect the absorbance of solution at 265nm (A_2).

4. Measurement of the solubility of solid dispersion samples   Precisely weigh 0.5g of solid dispersion of ibuprofen and PEG 6000 (calculated as ibuprofen, 0.05g), add 20ml of water, keep stirring for 5 mins and then filter the solution with microporous filter (0.45μm). Pipette 9ml of continuous filtrate and transfer to 10ml of volumetric flask, add 4% NaOH solution to 10ml, shake well. Detect the absorbance of solution at 265nm (A_3).

The concentration of ibuprofen in the three samples can be calculated by the above-mentioned regression equation.

5. DSC curves of ibuprofen DS samples   Take about 5.0mg of DS containing ibuprofen and PEG 6000, physical mixture of both materials (same quality ratio of ibuprofen to PEG 6000), raw ibuprofen and PEG 6000 with SD samples) and put them in an each small crucible provided by DSC company. The parameters of DSC are as followed: take α-Al_2O_3 as control; heating rate: 10℃/min; temperature range: 25~350℃; nitrogen environment. To observe the differences among three DSC curves from three samples, especially the alternations between DS and physical mixture.

【Notes】In the tests of the measurements of samples, stirring operation for each sample should be parallel and time of stirring is performed for 5 mins. Based on this, compare the solubility of different samples including raw ibuprofen, physical mixture, and ibuprofen SD.

 Results and Discussion

1. Results

(1) The resulted solubility of three samples including raw ibuprofen, physical mixture, and ibuprofen SD is recorded in the Table 14-1.

Table 14-1   The resulted solubility of three samples including raw ibuprofen, physical mixture, and ibuprofen SD

Sample	A Values	Solubility
Raw ibuprofen		
Physical mixture		
Ibuprofen SD		

(2) Draw the DSC curves of three samples including raw ibuprofen, physical mixture, and ibuprofen SD.

2. Discussions

(1) Compare the differences among three samples and provide a reasonable explain for the different points.

(2) In the tests of the measurements of samples, stirring time for each sample is performed for 5 mins. What is significance for the control of stirring time?

Questions

1. Whether PEG 6000 is needed to be crushed and sieved or not? Does its particle size affect the solubility of ibuprofen in physical mixtures and solid dispersions?

2. Sketch the principles of fast and sustained release of SD formulation.

3. The aging phenomenon of SD formulation always occur during the storage period. Hence what method could be developed to relieve or overcome the changes and improve the stability of formulation?

实验十五 包合物的制备及包合率的测定

实验目的

1. **掌握** β- 环糊精包合物的制备方法和包合率的测定方法。
2. **熟悉** β- 环糊精的性质及包合物的验证方法。

实验原理

包合物是一种形状、分子大小适宜的药物分子全部或部分包藏在另一种分子的空穴内形成的分子微型胶囊，由主分子和客分子组成。主分子即具有包合作用的外层分子，有较大的空穴结构，可以是单分子，也可以是多分子聚合而成。客分子是被包合到主分子空穴中的小分子物质。

目前药物制剂中常用的包合材料为环糊精，它为 6~12 个葡萄糖分子以 1, 4- 糖苷键连接而成的环状化合物，常见的环糊精为 α、β、γ- 环糊精，分别由 6、7、8 个葡萄糖分子构成，其中 β- 环糊精（β-CD）空穴内径 0.7~0.8nm，在水中的溶解度最小，易从水中析出，常作为制备包合物的材料。β- 环糊精溶解度随温度升高而增加（20、40、60、80、100℃下溶解度分别为 18.5、37、80、183、256g/L），因此，通过饱和水溶液法可获得药物的环糊精包合物，从而实现了提高一些药物的稳定性、增加溶解度和生物利用度、减少副作用和刺激性的目的，同时也具有使液态药物粉末化、掩盖药物不良臭味、防止药物挥发等作用。对于药物分子的一般要求如下：①分子量在 100~400 之间；②溶解度小于 10g/L；③分子中原子数不大于 5，且稠环数小于 5；④熔点低于 250℃。

环糊精包合物常用的制备方法有饱和水溶液法、研磨法、超声法、冷冻干燥法、喷雾干燥法等。本实验采用饱和水溶液法制备包合物，也称为重结晶法或共沉淀法，制备工艺流程如下：

β-CD + 水→饱和水溶液→滴加被包合物→磁力搅拌→冷藏→滤过→沉淀物干燥→即得

包合率直接影响包合物的质量，包合物中挥发油的回收参照《中国药典》挥发油测定法，采用水蒸气蒸馏法进行。

挥发油的包合率采用下式计算：

$$包合率 = [\ 包合物中挥发油回收量（ml）/挥发油加入量（ml）\ ] \times 100\%$$

除检查包合率外，可根据药物的性质选择不同的方法对包合物进行验证，判断是否形成包合物。常用的方法有显微镜法、薄层色谱法、热分析法、光谱法、X 射线衍射法、核磁共振法等。

实验器材

1. 仪器 差示扫描量热仪、恒温水浴锅、恒温磁力搅拌器、天平、冰箱、循环水真空泵、电热套、烘箱、挥发油提取器、烧杯、量筒、胶头滴管、锥形瓶、布氏漏斗、抽滤瓶、圆底烧瓶、冷凝管、容量瓶、硅胶 G 薄层板、层析缸、微量进样器或点样毛细管等。

2. **材料**　薄荷油、β-环糊精、无水乙醇、95% 乙醇、石油醚、乙酸乙酯、香草醛、浓硫酸、蒸馏水等。

实验方法

（一）薄荷油 β-环糊精包合物的制备

【处方】

薄荷油	2.0ml
β-环糊精	8.0g
蒸馏水	100ml

【制法】称取 β-环糊精（β-CD）8.0g，置于具塞锥形瓶中，加蒸馏水 100ml，加热使溶解，制得 β-环糊精饱和水溶液。保温 50℃，滴加薄荷油 2.0ml，恒温搅拌 2.5 小时，冷藏 24 小时，待沉淀完全后，抽滤。用无水乙醇 5ml 洗涤 3 次，至沉淀表面近无油渍，将包合物干燥，即得。

【性状】本品为白色干燥粉末。

【用途】为制剂过程的中间体。主要加入相应的片剂、颗粒剂、胶囊剂等固体制剂中发挥应有的治疗作用。

【注意事项】

（1）β-CD 溶解度在 25℃时为 1.79%，45℃时可增加至 3.1%，制备过程应控制好温度，尽可能在 45℃以下完成。

（2）包合温度、药物与 β-CD 的配比、包合时间等均影响包合率，制备时应按实验要求进行操作。

（3）难溶于水的药物也可用少量有机溶剂如乙醇等溶解后再加入 β-CD 的饱和水溶液中进行包合。

（4）包合完成后应降低温度使包合物从水中析出，并通过冷藏使包合物析出沉淀比较完全。

（二）包合率的测定

【方法】采用水蒸气蒸馏法。取制备好的包合物，精密称定重量，取约一半的包合物，精密称定重量，置圆底烧瓶中，加蒸馏水 300ml，连接挥发油提取器，蒸馏 2 小时以上，至油量不再增加，放置至室温，读取挥发油回收量（ml），计算挥发油包合率。

【注意事项】

（1）为计算包合率，一定要先明确实验取用的包合物中应含有的挥发油的量（计算时按包合率为 100% 计），包合物的取样一定要准确。

（2）本实验采用的是水蒸气蒸馏法回收包合物中的挥发油，蒸馏时间要适宜，要确保所取包合物中的挥发油尽可能全部回收，因此冷凝温度尽可能低。

（三）包合物的验证

1. **薄层色谱法**　取薄荷油 β-环糊精包合物 2g，加入 95% 乙醇 2ml，振摇 10 分钟，滤过，滤液为供试品溶液Ⅰ。另取包合物 2g 于圆底烧瓶中，加蒸馏水 100ml，连接挥发油提取器，提取挥发油，将提取得到的挥发油加 95% 乙醇 2ml 使溶解，作为供试品溶液Ⅱ。再取薄荷油 2 滴，加 95% 乙醇 2ml 使溶解，作为供试品溶液Ⅲ。吸取上述三种供试品溶液各 5μl，分别点于同一硅胶 G 薄层板上，以石油醚 - 乙酸乙酯（17∶3）为展开剂，展开，取出，晾干，喷以 1% 香草醛硫酸液，105℃烘至斑点显色清晰。

2. **差示扫描量热法**　各取 4.0~5.0mg 的薄荷油 -β- 环糊精包合物、薄荷油与 β- 环糊精的物理混合物（同包合物中比例）、β- 环糊精以及薄荷油，置于坩埚内。DSC 条件具体如下：以 α-Al$_2$O$_3$ 为参比物，升温速率为 10℃/min，升温范围：25~220℃（薄荷油升温 25~120℃），氮气保护。通过图谱吸热曲线变化观察各种样品，特别是薄荷油 -β- 环糊精包合物与薄荷油与 β- 环糊精的物理混合物的差异。

【注意事项】

（1）本实验验证包合过程是否实现了对薄荷挥发油的包合，为此制备了三种供试品溶液，预期实验结果是供试品溶液 I 未出现明显斑点，而供试品溶液 II 与供试品溶液 III 的斑点情况基本一致，进而证明包合物中有挥发油，且在 β-CD 的空穴中。

（2）展开前，需要预饱和 15~20 分钟。

（3）喷显色剂时要注意安全，不要使显色剂与人的皮肤接触，以免灼伤，一旦显色剂与人的皮肤接触，要及时用水冲洗。

实验结果与讨论

1. 薄荷油 β-CD 包合物的性状检查　薄荷油 β-CD 包合物的性状检查及包合率测定结果分别见表 15-1、表 15-2。

表 15-1　薄荷油 β-CD 包合物的性状检查结果

检查项目	检查结果
颜色	
性状	
嗅味	

表 15-2　薄荷油 β-CD 包合物包合率检查结果

检查项目	检查结果
包合物得到总量 /g	
包合物取样量 /g	
取样包合物中应含有的挥发油的量 /ml	
取样包合物中测得的挥发油的量 /ml	
包合率 /%	

2. 包合物的薄层色谱法验证　包合物的薄层色谱法验证结果见表 15-3。

表 15-3　薄荷油 β-CD 包合物薄层色谱法验证结果

供试液类型	斑点出现情况
供试液 I	
供试液 II	
供试液 III	
结论及分析	

3. 讨论　绘制薄荷油 β-CD 包合物、物理混合物、薄荷油及 β-CD 的 DSC 曲线，并分析实验结果。

思考题

1. β-环糊精包合物的制备方法有哪些?

2. 本实验为什么选用 β-环糊精为主分子? 它有什么特点?

3. β-环糊精包合物的作用有哪些?

（彭海生）

Lab. 15 Preparation of Cyclodextrin Complexes and Measurement of Inclusion Efficiency

 Experimental Objectives

1. To master the preparation process of β-cyclodextrin (β-CD) complexes and measurement of inclusion efficiency.

2. To be familiar with the features and identification methods of β-CD complexes.

 Experimental Principles

Inclusion complexes are molecular scale microcapsules, during which a molecule with suitable shape and size is partly or fully entrapped in an inner cavity of another molecule. The complexes are composed of host and guest molecules. Host molecule is either single molecule or macromolecule composed of multiple molecules which has a bigger cavity to room smaller molecule inside, called as guest molecule.

Nowadays, the commonly-used host materials in the medication are CD including α, β and γ three isoforms whose rings are composed of 6, 7 and 8 glucose residues, respectively. Among them, β-CD has interior diameter of cavity of 0.7~0.8nm and easily forms precipitate due to the lowest solubility in the water, hence has been becoming the most commonly-used host candidates. The solubility of β-CD will increase with increase of environmental temperature which solubilities are 18.5, 37, 80, 183 and 256g/L at 20, 40, 60, 80 and 100℃, respectively. Therefore, saturated aqueous solution method is used to prepare drug-β-CD complexes, thus improve the stability and solubility of active ingredients, increase the bioavailability of medication, as well as reduce side effects and irritation. The β-CD can entrap the liquid components and transform them into the powders, conceal the undesired odour, and prevent drug volatilization as well. The general requirements for guest molecules are as follows: ① molecular weigh with the range of 100~400 dalton; ② solubility less than 10g/L; ③ the number of atom in the molecule is not more than 5 and that of condensed ring is less than 5; and ④ the melting point below 250℃.

The commonly-used preparation methods for CD complexes are saturated aqueous solution, grinding, ultrasonic, freeze-drying and spray drying method, etc. Here, saturated aqueous solution method, also called as recrystallization or co-precipitation method, is used to prepare the CD complexes and the process are as under:

β-CD+water → saturated aqueous solution of CD → slowly dripping the entrapped active ingredients → magnetic stirring → refrigerate → filter → dry the sediment → obtain the CD complexes

Inclusion efficiency (IE) of CD complexes directly affects the quality of products and recovery of volatile oil from inclusion compound according to the determination method of volatile oil in *Chinese Pharmacopoeia* and is determined by the method of steam distillation.

110

Inclusion efficiency of CD complexes can be calculated as under:

IE= [the amount recovered from complexes (ml) / theoretical amount (ml)]× 100%

Except that IE is needed to evaluated, the identification of CD complexes, based on the properties of drug, can be performed by some methods including light microscopy, thin layer chromatography (TLC), thermal analysis, spectroscopy, X-ray diffraction, and nuclear magnetic resonance, etc.

 Equipments and Materials

1. Equipments Differential scanning calorimetry (DSC), constant temperature water bath, constant temperature magnetic stirrer, electronic balance, refrigerator, circulating water vacuum pump, electric heating sleeve, oven, volatile oil extractor, beaker, measuring cylinder, rubber-capped dropper, conical flask, Buchner funnel, suction flask, round bottom flask, condenser, volumetric flask, silica gel G thin layer plate, chromatography cylinder, microinjector or sampling capillary, etc.

2. Materials Peppermint oil, β-CD, anhydrous ethanol, 95% ethanol solution, petroleum ether, ethyl acetate, vanillin, concentrated sulfuric acid, distilled water, etc.

 Experimental Methods

I. Preparation of Peppermint Oil-β-CD Complexes

【Formula】

Peppermint oil	2.0ml
β-CD	8.0g
Distilled water	100ml

【Procedure】Weigh 8.0g of β-CD and put it into the conical flask with a top, add 100ml of distilled water, heat it to dissolve, obtain the β-CD saturated solution. Keep the temperature of solution at 50℃, slowly drip 2.0ml of peppermint oil, keep stirring for 2.5 hours at the same temperature and then refrigerate for 24 hours to completely obtain precipitate of complexes, filter the precipitate using a suction apparatus with a vaccum and wash the precipitate with 5.0ml of anhydrous ethanol three times near to no oil left on the surface of the precipitate, dry the complexes and obtain it.

【Description】Peppermint Oil-β-CD complexes are white dry powders.

【Application】An intermediate for a given preparation such as tablets, granules, capsules, and other solid preparations to play their due therapeutic role.

【Notes】

(1) The solubility of β-CD at 25℃ is 1.79% while that of β-CD would increase to 3.1% at 45℃. Thus the temperature of the solution, during the formation of β-CD complexes, should be controlled well and finish this process as far as possible below 45℃.

(2) The factors such as inclusion temperature, the ratio of amount of active ingredients to that of β-CD, the length of time taken for inclusion, etc all affect inclusion efficiency of peppermint Oil-β-CD complexes. Thus all operation should follow the requirements of tests.

(3) For water poorly soluble molecules, small amount of organic solvent such as ethanol can be used to dissolve these drugs and transfer the solution to β-CD saturated solution and finish the operation.

(4) After inclusion, decrease the temperature of inclusion complexes solution to form precipitate and refrigerate the samples to improve the recovery rate of inclusion complexes.

II. Measurement of Inclusion Efficiency

【Procedure】Steam distillation method: The resulted peppermint Oil-β-CD complexes, take one half of samples, precisely weigh, transfer them to round bottom flask, add 300ml of distilled water into the flask, then connected with volatile oil extractor, extract 2 hours to no increase of amount of volatile oil, put the flask aside at room temperature. Read the recovery amount of oil (ml) and calculate the inclusion efficiency of peppermint Oil-β-CD complexes.

【Notes】

(1) To accurately calculate the inclusion efficiency, the theoretical amount of peppermint oil in the complexes should be evaluated before extraction (IE calculated as, 100%), thus precisely sampling peppermint oil-β-CD complexes is needed.

(2) Steam distillation method is here used to extract the peppermint oil, thus distillation timing should be suitable to recover all the oil and condensation temperature as low as possible.

III. Identification of β-CD Complexes

1. TLC method: Take 2.0g of peppermint oil-β-CD complexes, add 2.0ml of 95% ethanol solution, shake for 10 mins, and filter; take the resulted filtrate as test solution I. Take another 2.0g of peppermint oil-β-CD complexes and transfer to round bottom flask, add 100ml distilled water to the flask, assemble volatile oil extractor and extract the oil; added 2.0ml of 95% ethanol solution to dissolve the resulted oil, taken it as test solution II. Take two drops of peppermint oil and add 95% ethanol solution to dissolve it, taken it as test solution II. Pipette 5.0μl of above-mentioned three solutions, respectively point it on the same silica gel G thin layer plate; then take the mixture of petroleum ether and ethyl acetate (17:3) as developer and develop the samples; take it out, dry it and spray with 1% vanillin sulfuric acid, afterwards the plates is put into the oven at 105℃ to heat until the spots are clear.

2. DSC method: Take about 4.0~5.0mg of peppermint oil-β-CD complexes, physical mixture of both materials (same quality ratio of peppermint oil to β-CD), peppermint oil and β-CD) and put them in an each small crucible provided by DSC company. The parameters of DSC are as followed: take $α-Al_2O_3$ as control; heating rate: 10℃/min; temperature range: 25~120℃; nitrogen environment. To observe the differences among four DSC curves from three samples, especially the alternations between peppermint oil-β-CD complexes and physical mixture.

【Notes】

(1) To identify the formation of peppermint oil-β-CD complexes, three test solutions are prepared. As expected, there would be no evident spots of peppermint oil on the plate pointed with test solution I whereas there would be spots of the oil at the same positions of two plates pointed with test solution II and III, respectively, which verify that there is peppermint oil in the interior cavity of β-CD complexes.

(2) Before development, the environment of chromatography cylinder should need presaturation with developers for 15~20 mins to improve results of development.

(3) When spaying the chromogenic reagent, pay carefully attention to rules of safe operation; and do not make any agents contact with human skin to avoid burns. Once the developer contacts with human skin, wash it with water in time.

 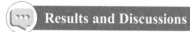 **Results and Discussions**

1. Description of peppermint oil-β-CD complexes Description and IE of peppermint oil-β-CD complexes should be listed in the Table 15–1 and Table 15–2.

Table 15–1 Description of peppermint oil-β-CD complexes

Items	Results
Color	
Appearance	
Odour	

Table 15–2 IE of peppermint oil-β-CD complexes

Items	Results
Total amount of peppermint oil-β-CD complexes/g	
Amount of peppermint oil-β-CD complexes taken/g	
Theoretical amount of peppermint oil in the complexes taken/ml	
Detected amount of peppermint oil in the complexes taken/ml	
IE/%	

2. Identification of peppermint oil-β-CD complexes by TLC　　The results of identification of peppermint oil-β-CD complexes by TLC should be provided in the Table 15–3.

Table 15–3 Identification of peppermint oil-β-CD complexes by TLC

Test solution	Spots
I	
II	
III	
Conclusion and analysis	

3. Discussion　　Draw the DSC curves of four samples including peppermint oil-β-CD complexes, physical mixture, peppermint oil and β-CD. And then analyze experimental results.

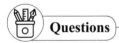 **Questions**

1. Please list all preparation methods of β-CD complexes?
2. Why β-CD is used as host molecules in this experiment and what features it has?
3. What are the functions of β-CD complexes?

PPT

实验十六 微囊的制备及质量评价

实验目的

1. **掌握** 复凝聚法制备微囊的原理、工艺及操作要点。
2. **熟悉** 微囊的成囊条件、影响因素及质量控制方法。

实验原理

微囊是用天然、合成或半合成高分子材料作为囊膜将固体或液体药物包囊而形成的微小胶囊，粒径 1~250μm。根据需要可将微囊进一步制成散剂、胶囊剂、片剂、注射剂、软膏剂、凝胶剂等剂型。

常见的微囊制备方法有三种：物理化学法、物理机械法、化学法。可根据药物的性质、囊材的性质、微囊的粒径、释放和靶向要求、设备等条件选择不同的制备方法。凝聚法分单凝聚法和复凝聚法，后者更为常用。复凝聚法是采用带相反电荷的两种高分子材料作为囊材，在一定条件下交联且与药物凝聚成囊的方法。该法操作简便、容易掌握，适合于难溶性固体药物和液体药物微囊。

微囊的囊心物可以是固体药物，也可以是液体药物。除药物外，还可酌情加入附加剂：稳定剂、稀释剂、增塑剂、促进剂与阻滞剂。

明胶和阿拉伯胶是最常用的天然高分子材料。明胶是胶原蛋白的水解产物，根据水解方法的不同，明胶有酸法明胶（A 型）和碱法明胶（B 型）之分。A 型明胶的等电点在 pH 7~9，B 型明胶的等电点在 pH 4.8~5.2。明胶是两性蛋白质，在水溶液中分子含有—NH_2、—$COOH$ 及相应的解离基团—NH_3^+、—COO^-。所含正负离子的多少受介质 pH 的影响。pH 较低时—NH_3^+ 的数量多于—COO^-；反之，—COO^- 的数量多于—NH_3^+。两种电荷相等时的 pH 为等电点。当 pH 在等电点以上时明胶带负电，当 pH 在等电点以下时明胶带正电。两种明胶在成囊性能上无明显差异，可生物降解，几乎无抗原性，通常可根据药物对酸碱性的要求选用 A 型 B 型明胶。阿拉伯胶在水溶液中分子链上含有—$COOH$ 和—COO^-，因此，阿拉伯胶仅带负电荷。

复凝聚法（complex coacervation）制备微囊的原理：将溶液的 pH 调至明胶的等电点以下使明胶带正电荷（pH 4.0~4.5 时明胶带正电荷最多），阿拉伯胶带负电荷。由于正、负电荷相互吸引交联形成络合物，溶解度降低而凝聚成囊，加水稀释，甲醛交联固化，用水洗至无甲醛味，即得微囊。

囊材品种、胶液浓度、成囊温度、搅拌速度及 pH 等因素，对成囊过程和成品质量有重要影响，制备时应从严控制成囊条件。

微囊质量评价的项目包括：外观形态、粒径、载药量、包封率、微囊中药物的释放速率、有机溶剂残留量等。

实验器材

1. **仪器**　天平、组织捣碎机、磁力加热搅拌器、水浴锅、烘箱、抽滤装置、2号筛、显微镜、广泛pH试纸、精密pH试纸、烧杯（500、250及50ml）、量筒、载玻片、盖玻片、擦镜纸、玻璃棒、冰浴等。

2. **材料**　液状石蜡、A型明胶、阿拉伯胶、37%甲醛溶液、10%醋酸溶液、20%氢氧化钠溶液、蒸馏水等。

实验方法

（一）液状石蜡微囊的制备

【处方】

液状石蜡	6ml
A型明胶	5g
阿拉伯胶	5g
37%甲醛溶液	2.5ml
10%醋酸溶液	适量
20%氢氧化钠溶液	适量
蒸馏水	适量

【制法】

（1）5%明胶溶液的配制　取明胶5g，用蒸馏水适量浸泡溶胀，微热溶解，加蒸馏水至100ml，搅匀，50℃保温备用。

（2）5%阿拉伯胶溶液的配制　取蒸馏水80ml置烧杯中，加阿拉伯胶粉末5g，加热至80℃左右，轻轻搅拌使溶解，加蒸馏水至100ml。

（3）液状石蜡乳的制备　取液状石蜡6ml和5%阿拉伯胶溶液100ml置组织捣碎机中，乳化5分钟，即得液状石蜡乳，备用。

（4）乳剂镜检　取液状石蜡乳一滴，置载玻片上，镜检，绘制乳剂外观形态图。

（5）混合　将液状石蜡乳倒入1000ml烧杯中，置50~55℃水浴，加入5%明胶溶液，轻轻搅拌使混合均匀。

（6）微囊的制备　在不断搅拌下，滴加10%醋酸溶液于混合液中，调pH在3.8~4.0。

（7）微囊的固化　在不断搅拌下，将400ml蒸馏水（30℃）加至微囊液中，将含微囊液的烧杯自50~55℃水浴取下，不停搅拌，使之自然冷却，待温度降至32~35℃时，加入冰块，继续搅拌至温度降至10℃以下，加入37%甲醛溶液2.5ml（用蒸馏水稀释一倍），搅拌15分钟，再用20%NaOH溶液调整pH至8~9，继续搅拌20分钟，观察至有析出为止，静置使微囊沉降。

（8）镜检　在显微镜下观察微囊的形态，绘制外观形态图。

【性状】本品为白色或类白色颗粒。

【注意事项】

（1）实验所用的水为蒸馏水或去离子水，以避免水中的离子影响凝聚过程。

（2）配制5%明胶溶液时，应先使明胶充分溶胀至溶解（必要时加热），以免结块不易溶解。

（3）微囊的制备过程中，始终伴随搅拌，搅拌速度要适中，搅拌速度太慢微囊易粘连，搅拌速度过快微囊易变形。搅拌速度以泡沫产生最少为佳，必要时可加入几滴戊醇或辛醇消泡。固化前勿停止搅拌，防止微囊粘连。

（4）用10%醋酸溶液调pH时，应逐滴加入，特别是当pH接近4时应更小心，并随时取样在显微镜下观察微囊的形成。

（5）实验过程中注意温度的控制。当温度接近凝固点时，微囊容易粘连，故加30℃、400ml蒸馏水的目的是稀释凝聚囊，以改善微囊形态。应搅拌至10℃以下后再加入甲醛，有利于交联固化。

（6）采用复凝聚法制备微囊时，应在50℃左右将其烘干，不宜室温或低温干燥，防止其粘连结块。

（二）质量评价

【外观】观察微囊的外观、颜色。

【形态】用光学显微镜、扫描或透射电子显微镜观察微囊外观形态，并绘图。

【粒径】用校正过的带目镜测微仪的光学显微镜测定微囊大小。亦可用库尔特计数器测定微囊大小及粒度分布。

实验结果与讨论

1. **微囊的外观** 观察并记录微囊的外观和颜色。

2. **微囊与乳剂的形态** 取少许湿微囊，加适量蒸馏水分散，盖上盖玻片（注意排除气泡），显微镜镜检，绘制微囊的外观形态图；与显微镜下的乳剂形态进行对比。

3. **微囊大小的测定** 取少许湿微囊，加适量蒸馏水分散，盖上盖玻片（注意排除气泡），用带刻度标尺（已校正每格的 μm 数）的显微镜镜检，在显微镜下观察并测定200个微囊的粒径，按式（16-1）计算微囊的算数平均径 d_{av}。

$$d_{av} = \sum (nd) / \sum n = (n_1d_1 + n_2d_2 + \cdots + n_nd_n) / (n_1 + n_2 + \cdots + n_n) \tag{16-1}$$

式中，n_1，n_2，$\cdots$，n_n 为具有粒径 d_1，d_1，$\cdots$，d_n 的粒子数。

根据微囊粒径测定结果，分析影响微囊大小的因素及控制方法。

4. **分析** 根据微囊粒径测定结果，分析影响微囊大小的因素及控制方法。

思考题

1. 简述复凝聚法制备微囊的工艺过程及操作要点。

2. 药物微囊化有哪些优点？

3. 试比较单凝聚法和复凝聚法制备微囊的异同点。

（陈新梅）

Lab. 16 Preparation and Quality Evaluation of Microcapsules

 Experimental Objectives

1. To master the principle, preparation process and key operations of preparation of microcapsules using complex coacervation method.

2. To be familiar with the microcapsules-forming conditions, influencing factors and the quality control methods.

 Experimental Principles

Microcapsules are a kind of microscale capsules that are made of the natural, the semi-synthetic or the synthetic polymers, encapsulated the solid or liquid drugs inside. The particle size is 1~250μm. The microcapsules can be further prepared into powders, capsules, tablets, injections, ointments, gels and other dosage forms as required.

There are three common methods to prepare the microcapsules, including physicochemical, physicomechanical and chemical methods. Selecting preparation method depends on the properties of the drugs and the polymers, the size of the microcapsules, the requirements of the release rate and target capability and the equipments available. The coacervation method, that belongs to the physicochemical method, is often be used to prepare the microcapsules. There are two kinds of coacervation methods, single coacervation and complex coacervation, the latter of which is more often used. The principle of the complex coacervation method is attractive forces of some hydrophilic polymers with opposite charges to form microcapsules loaded with drugs, and then conjugation of these polymers by some linker in a reacting condition to stablize the drug-loaded capsules. The complex coacervation method is simple and easy to master, which is suitable for insoluble and liquid drugs.

The drug in the microcapsules can be the solid or liquid substance. Besides, additives such as stabilizer, diluent, plasticizer, accelerator and blocker, can also be loaded into microcapsule according to the requirements.

Gelatin and Arabic gum are the most commonly used polymers. Gelatin hydrolyzed by acid or basic can be divided into acid-hydrolyzed gelatin(type A) and alkali-hydrolyzed one(type B). The isoelectric point of gelatin A or B is in the range of pH 7~9 or pH 4.8~5.2, respectively. Gelatin, an amphoteric protein, containing —NH$_2$ and —COOH group dissociates to form group of —NH$_3^+$ and —COO$^-$. The amount of the positive and negative irons in the gelatin is affected by the pH of the medium. When pH is lower than isoelectric point (IP), the amount of —NH$_3^+$ is more than —COO$^-$, vice versa. When the amount of positive and negative is equal, the pH value is the isoelectric point. When the pH value is bigger than IP, the gelatin is negatively charged. When the pH value is below the isoelectric point,

117

the gelatin carries positive charges, vice versa. There are no obvious differences between the two kinds of gelatins in the performance of drug-encapsulating. They are biodegradable and have almost no antigencity. Generally, selecting A-type or B-type gelatin is depended on acid base property of the drug. Arabic gum only contains —COOH and —COO⁻ group on the molecular chain in aqueous solution, thus, Arabic gum is only negatively charged.

The principle of the complex coacervation method is that: Adjust the pH value of solution to below the IP of the gelatin, which makes gelatin positively charged(gelatin has the most positive charges at the pH value 4.0~4.5), while Arabic gum is negatively charged simultaneously. As the positive and negative charges attract each other and cross link to form a complex. The solubility of the complex is reduced and condensed into microcapsules. Diluted the solution containing the microcapsules with water, cross linded and solidified with formaldehyde and washed with water until it is free from formaldehyde, and then the microcapsules can be obtained.

During the process of preparing the microcapsules, the conditions should be controlled strictly for the reason that many factors such as the type of the polymers, the solution concentration of the gelatin or Arabic gum, the temperature, the speed of the mixing and the pH value have an important influence to the formation and the quality of the microcapsules.

The quality evaluation of microcapsules includes: Appearance and morphology, particle size, drug loading, encapsulation rate, release speed of the drug from the microcapsules and the residual of the organic solution etc.

Equipments and Materials

1. Equipments   Analytical balance(scale), tissue masher, magnetic stirrer, constant temperature water bather, oven, filter with vacuum, No.2 sieve, microscope, broad pH test paper, accurate pH test paper, beaker(500, 250 and 50ml), cylinder, glass slide, cover slip, lens paper, glass rod, ice bath, etc.

2. Materials   Liquid paraffin, gelatin A, Arabic gum, 37% formaldehyde solution, 10% acetic acid solution, 20% sodium hydroxide solution, distilled water, etc.

Experimental Methods

I. Preparation of Liquid Paraffin Loaded Microcapsules

【Formula】

Liquid paraffin	6ml
Gelatin A	5g
Arabic gum	5g
37% Formaldehyde solution	2.5ml
10% Acetic acid	q.s.
20% Sodium hydroxide solution	q.s.
Distilled water	q.s.

【Procedure】

(1) Preparation of 5% Gelatin solution: Take 5g of gelatin, soak it in the distilled water for swelling. Slightly heat the solution to dissolve gelatin and add distilled water to 100ml, homogenize, keep warm at 50℃ for standby.

(2) Preparation of 5% Arabic gum solution: Take 80ml of distilled water and put it in the beaker. Add 5g Arabic gum power into the water and heat mixture about 80℃, keep stirring gently to solve it and add the distilled water to 100ml.

(3) Preparation of liquid paraffin emulsion: Take 6ml of liquid paraffin and 100ml of 5% Arabic gum solution into the tissue masher, emulsify them for 5 minutes and then get the liquid paraffin emulsion for standby.

(4) Microscopic inspection: Take a drop of liquid paraffin emulsion, put it on the slide and observe it with the microscope. Draw the appearance and the morphology of the emulsion.

(5) Mixing: Transfer the liquid emulsion into the 1000ml beaker, place it in the water bather (50~55℃). Add 5% gelatin solution and stir it gently to mix evenly.

(6) Preparation of microcapsules: Add 10% acetic acid solution to the mixture under the constant agitation. Adjust the pH value to the range of 3.8~4.0.

(7) Solidification of microcapsules: Add 400ml of distilled water (30℃) to the microcapsule solution under the constant agitation. Take the beaker containing the microcapsule solution out from the water bather at 50~55℃ and keep stirring to make it cool naturally. Add the ice when the temperature drops to 32~35℃ and continue to stir until the temperature drops to below 10℃. Add 37% formaldehyde solution of 2.5ml (dilute with distilled water) and keep stirring for 15 minutes. Adjust the pH value to 8~9 with 10% NaOH solution. Continue to stir for 20 minutes and observe until precipitation phenomena occurred. Let it stand to make the microcapsules settle down.

(8) Microscope inspection: Observe the appearance under the microscope and draw the morphology of the microscopes.

【Description】This product is white or similar white particles.

【Notes】

(1) The distilled water or deionized water should be used to avoid the condensation influence from the ion in the water.

(2) When prepared 5% gelatin solution, the gelatin should be fully expanded to dissolved(Heated if necessary) to avoid caking.

(3) During the preparation of the microcapsules, keep moderately stirring is necessary to avoid capsules adhesion in lower stirring speed and capsules deformation in high stirring speed. The optimized stirring speed is adjust to minimize the foam production. If necessary, a few drops of amyl alcohol or octanol can be added to defoam. Don't stop mixing before solidification and decrease the adhesion of microcapsules.

(4) When adjusted pH value with 10% acetic acid, it should be added drop by drop, especially when the pH value is close to 4. Samples should be continuously taken to observe the formation of the microcapsules using the microscope.

(5) Pay attention to the temperature control during the experiment. When the temperature is close to the solidification point, the microcapsules are easy to adhere. Thus, add 400ml of distilled water at 30℃ to dilute the microcapsules solution so as to improve the morphology of the microcapsules. Keep stirring until temperature of the solution reach to 10℃, then add formaldehyde to facilitate the solidification of capsule.

(6) When microcapsules are prepared by complex coacervation method, they should be dried at around 50℃, not at room temperature or lower temperature so as to prevent sticking and caking.

II. Quality Evaluation

【Appearance】Observe the appearance and the color of the microcapsules.

【Morphology】Observe the appearance and morphology with an optical microscope, a scan electronic microscope or a transmission electronic microscope and draw the picture.

【Particle size】Measure the microcapsules size with an optical microscope which has a calibrated eyepiece micrometer. Kurt counter can also be used to detect the size and the size distribution of the microcapsules.

 Results and Discussion

1. Appearance: Observe and record the appearance and color of the microcapsules.

2. Morphology of the microcapsules and the emulsion:Take a little wet microcapsules and add some distilled water to disperse them. Cover with cover slip (exclude the bubbles) and observation under a microscope. Draw the picture of the microcapsules and compare them with the emulsions under a microscope.

3. Determination of the size:Take a little wet microcapsules and add some distilled water to disperse them. Cover with cover slip (exclude the bubbles) and observe under a microscope which has scale (μm number per lattice has been calibrated). Observe and detect the size of 200 microcapsules and calculate the average size the microcapsules d_{av} according to the formula below.

$$d_{av} = \sum (nd) / \sum n = (n_1 d_1 + n_2 d_2 + \cdots + n_n d_n) / (n_1 + n_2 + \cdots + n_n) \tag{16-1}$$

In the above formula:$n_1, n_2, \cdots, n_n$ is particle number, $d_1, d_2, \cdots, d_n$ is particle size.

4. Analyze: Analyze the influencing factors and controlling methods of the microcapsules size according to the detecting results.

 Questions

1. Introduce the process and the key point of preparing the microcapsules using the complex coacervation method.

2. What are the advantages of drug microcapsulaiton?

3. Compare the similarities and differences between the single coacervation and complex coacervation methods to prepare the microcapsules.

实验十七 脂质体的制备及包封率测定

实验目的

1. **掌握** 薄膜分散法制备脂质体的工艺；阳离子交换树脂法测定脂质体包封率的方法。
2. **熟悉** 脂质体的形成原理及主动载药与被动载药的含义。

实验原理

　　脂质体是指药物包封于类脂质双分子层结构中所制成的超微型封闭囊状载体。磷脂是构成脂质体的主要成分，其分子结构中有两条较长的疏水碳氢链（非极性尾部）和亲水的磷酸基团（极性头部）。将适量磷脂加至水中，其分子会产生自组装定向排列，疏水碳氢链彼此缔合为双分子层，而亲水基团在双分子层的两侧面向内、外水相，以构成脂质体。为改善脂质体性能，常需加入胆固醇、十八胺、磷脂酸等附加剂。胆固醇与磷脂混合使用，可调节脂质体膜的通透性，提高其稳定性。十八胺、磷脂酸则可通过改变脂质体表面的电荷性质，以改善其包封率、稳定性及体内分布等性能。

　　脂质体的制法根据载药机制的不同，可分为主动载药、被动载药两大类。主动载药是先制备含有浓缩离子或分子的空白脂质体，再与另一离子或化合物溶液孵育，利用其内外水相间形成的浓度梯度进行载药，包括 K^+-Na^+ 梯度、H^+ 梯度（即 pH 梯度），适用于包封率极易受包封条件影响的两亲性药物脂质体的制备。被动载药是先将药物溶于水相或有机相中，再选择适宜方法以制得含药脂质体，是采用最多的一类方法，适用于脂溶性且与磷脂膜亲和力高的药物脂质体的制备。

　　脂质体的评价主要包括形态、粒径、表面电性、泄漏率、包封率、载药量等指标。包封率是评价脂质体制备过程的重要指标，主要受脂质体的膜材组成、水相体积、数目以及药物与磷脂膜的作用力、药脂比等因素影响，可采用阳离子交换树脂、分子筛、超滤等方法测定。阳离子交换树脂法是利用离子交换作用，将荷正电的未包进脂质体中游离药物吸附除去，而包封于脂质体中药物不被树脂吸附以达到两者分离，再分别测定药物含量，即可计算其包封率。

实验器材

　　1. **仪器** 烧瓶、烧杯、容量瓶、量筒、移液管、玻璃棉、针筒注射器（5ml）、微量注射器（100μl）、微孔滤膜（0.8μm）、电子天平、旋转蒸发仪、水浴锅、磁力搅拌器、光学显微镜、紫外-可见分光光度计等。
　　2. **材料** 枸橼酸、枸橼酸钠、大豆磷脂（注射用）、胆固醇、无水乙醇、磷酸氢二钠、磷酸二氢钠、盐酸小檗碱、碳酸氢钠、732 型阳离子交换树脂、95% 乙醇等。

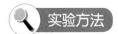 实验方法

（一）空白脂质体的制备

【处方】

大豆磷脂（注射用）	1.8g
胆固醇	0.6g
无水乙醇	4ml
枸橼酸缓冲液	适量

【制法】

（1）枸橼酸缓冲液（pH 3.8）的配制　称取枸橼酸 10.5g 和枸橼酸钠 7.0g 置于 1000ml 量瓶中，加水溶解并稀释至刻度，混匀，即得。取 60ml，置于小烧杯内，55~60℃水浴中保温，待用。

（2）称取处方量磷脂、胆固醇于 100ml 烧瓶中，加无水乙醇 4ml，55~60℃水浴，搅拌使溶解，于旋转蒸发仪上旋转，使磷脂/胆固醇的乙醇液在壁上成膜，减压除去乙醇，制得脂质膜。

（3）将"（1）"中预热的枸橼酸缓冲液加至"（2）"中，转动下 55~60℃水化 10 分钟，取出移至烧杯内，置磁力搅拌器上，室温下搅拌 20~30 分钟。如溶液体积减少，可补加蒸馏水至 60ml，混匀，即得。

【注意事项】

（1）实验过程中禁用明火。

（2）磷脂和胆固醇的乙醇溶液应澄清，不能在水浴中放置过长时间。

（3）制备脂质膜时，应尽量使其薄而均匀。

（4）水化时，要充分保证所有脂质水化，不得存在脂质块。

（二）盐酸小檗碱被动载药脂质体的制备

【处方】

大豆磷脂（注射用）	1.2g
胆固醇	0.4g
无水乙醇	4ml
盐酸小檗碱溶液（1mg/ml）	60ml

【制法】

（1）磷酸盐缓冲液（PBS，pH 5.8）的配制　称取磷酸氢二钠 0.37g 与磷酸二氢钠 2.0g，加蒸馏水适量，溶解并稀释至 1000ml，混匀，即得。

（2）盐酸小檗碱溶液的配制　称取适量盐酸小檗碱，用 PBS 配成浓度为 1mg/ml（60℃水浴加热溶解）的溶液。

（3）按处方量称取磷脂、胆固醇置 100ml 烧瓶中，加无水乙醇 4ml，余下操作除将枸橼酸缓冲液换成盐酸小檗碱溶液外，同"空白脂质体的制备"项下方法制备，即得。

（三）盐酸小檗碱主动载药脂质体的制备

【处方】

空白脂质体	2ml
碳酸氢钠溶液	0.1ml
盐酸小檗碱溶液（3mg/ml）	1ml

【制法】

（1）盐酸小檗碱溶液的配制　称取适量盐酸小檗碱，用 PBS 配成浓度为 3mg/ml（60℃水浴加热溶解）的溶液。

（2）碳酸氢钠溶液（pH 7.8）的配制　称取 $NaHCO_3$ 50g，置于 1000ml 量瓶中，加水溶解并稀释至 1000ml，混匀，即得。

（3）主动载药　移取空白脂质体混悬液（事先通过 0.8μm 微孔滤膜两遍整粒）2ml、盐酸小檗碱溶液 1ml、$NaHCO_3$ 溶液 0.5ml，在振摇下依次加于 10ml 西林瓶中，混匀，加塞，60℃水浴中保温孵育 15 分钟，随后立即用冷水降温，终止载药，即得。

【注意事项】

（1）主动载药过程中，加药顺序不能颠倒，边加边摇，以确保混合均匀，使体系中各部位的梯度一致。

（2）水浴保温时，应注意随时轻摇（或每隔 1 分钟，手摇 20 秒），但注意以保证体系均匀为度，无需剧烈振摇。

（3）冷却终止载药过程中也应轻摇。

（四）形态观察及粒径测定

取样，在油镜下观察脂质体的形态，画出脂质体结构，记录脂质体的最大粒径和最多粒径；将所得脂质体液体通过 0.8μm 微孔滤膜两遍整粒，再于油镜下观察脂质体形态，画出所见脂质体结构，记录脂质体最大粒径和最多粒径。

（五）包封率的测定

1. 阳离子交换树脂分离柱制备　称取已活化好的阳离子交换树脂适量，装于底部已垫有少量玻璃棉的 5ml 注射器筒中，加入 PBS 水化阳离子交换树脂，自然滴尽 PBS，即得。

2. 柱分离度考察

（1）盐酸小檗碱与空白脂质体混合液的制备　精密量取盐酸小檗碱溶液（3mg/ml）0.1ml，置于小试管中，加入 0.2ml 空白脂质体混悬液，混匀，即得。

（2）空白溶剂的配制　取乙醇（95%）6ml，置 10ml 量瓶中，加 PBS 稀释至刻度，摇匀，即得。

（3）对照品溶液的制备　精密移取（1）项所得混合液 0.1ml 置 10ml 量瓶中，加入 95% 乙醇 6ml，振摇使之溶解澄明，再加 PBS 稀释至刻度，摇匀，过滤，弃去初滤液，取续滤液 4ml 于 10ml 量瓶中，加（2）项下空白溶剂稀释至刻度，摇匀，即得。

（4）样品溶液的制备　精密移取（1）项所得混合液 0.1ml 上样于阳离子交换树脂柱（柱长 1cm）顶部，待顶部液体消失后，放置 5 分钟，仔细加入 2~3ml PBS（注意不能将柱顶部的树脂冲散）进行洗脱，收集洗脱液于 10ml 量瓶中，加入 95% 乙醇 6ml，振摇使之溶解澄明，再加 PBS 稀释至刻度，摇匀，过滤，弃取初滤液，取续滤液即得。

（5）吸收度测定及柱分离度的计算　以空白溶剂为对照，在 345nm 波长处分别测定样品溶液与对照品溶液的吸收度，按式（17-1）计算柱分离度。

$$柱分离度 = 1 - A_样 / (A_对 \times 2.5) \tag{17-1}$$

式中，$A_样$ 为样品溶液的吸收度；$A_对$ 为对照品溶液的吸收度；2.5 为对照品溶液相对于样品溶液的稀释倍数；柱分离度值要求大于 0.90。

3. 包封率的测定　精密移取盐酸小檗碱脂质体 0.1ml 两份，一份置于 10ml 量瓶中，按"2.柱分离度考察"项下（3）进行操作，另一份置于分离柱顶部，按"2.柱分离度考察"项下（4）进行操作，所得溶液分别于 345nm 波长处测定吸收度，按式（17-2）计算包封率。

$$包封率 = A_2 / (A_1 \times 2.5) \times 100\% \tag{17-2}$$

式中，A_2 为分离后脂质体中盐酸小檗碱的吸收度；A_1 为未分离盐酸小檗碱脂质体中盐酸小檗碱的总吸收度；2.5 为未分离脂质体相对于分离后脂质体的稀释倍数。

实验结果与讨论

1. 实验结果

（1）拍摄显微镜下各脂质体样品的图片，并进行描述。

（2）记录测定的脂质体最大粒径和最多粒径（表17-1）。

（3）记录测定的柱分离度与包封率（表17-1）。

表 17-1　脂质体形态与粒径的测定结果

脂质体样品	形态	最大粒径 /μm	最多粒径 /μm	柱分离度	包封率 /%
空白脂质体					——
盐酸小檗碱被动载药脂质体					
盐酸小檗碱主动载药脂质体					

2. 讨论

（1）对比分析主动载药法与被动载药法制备盐酸小檗碱脂质体的优劣及其原因。

（2）与其他小组的实验结果进行对比，是否存在差异？若存在明显差异，请分析原因。

思考题

1. 脂质体形成的主要影响因素有哪些？

2. 脂质体主动包载和被动包载药物的原理及其特点是什么？

3. 如何提高脂质体对药物的包封率？

（谢兴亮）

Lab. 17　Preparation of Liposomes and Determination of Encapsulation Efficiency

 Experimental Objectives

1. To master the technology of preparing liposome by thin film dispersion method and determination method of encapsulation efficiency of vesicles by cation-exchange resin.

2. To be familiar with the formation principle of liposomes and the meaning of active loading and passive loading of drug into vesicles.

 Experimental Principles

Liposome is a kind of nano-, or microscale enclosed vesicular carrier with lipid bilayer structures loaded with drugs. Phospholipid is the main component of vesicles, which has two hydrophobic hydrocarbon chains (non-polar tails) and hydrophilic phosphate group (polar head). When an appropriate amount of phospholipid is added into water, their molecules produce oriented arrangement in a self-assembled manner. In brief, hydrophobic hydrocarbon chains of phospholipid associate with each other to form the main structure of bilayers while hydrophilic groups face the inner aqueous phases and outside aqueous environment on both sides of the bilayer, resulting to the self-assembled liposomes. In order to improve the performance of liposomes, cholesterol, octadecylamine, phosphatidic acid, and other additives are often added. The addition of cholesterol and phospholipids adjust the permeability of the liposome membrane and its stability. Octadecylamine and phosphatidic acid are used to optimize the encapsulation efficiency, stability, and the *in vivo* distribution by changing the charge properties of liposome surface.

According to the different loading mechanism, the method of drug loading of liposomes can be categorized as active drug loading and passive one. Active drug loading is to prepare liposomes containing a concentrated ion or molecules but drug (blank liposomes), then remove same ingredients from external aqueous phase; and incubate with another ion or compound solution and form concentration gradients between its internal and external aqueous phases to load drug, including K^+-Na^+ gradient, H^+ gradient (i.e. pH gradient), which is suitable for the preparation of amphiphilic drug-loaded liposomes whose encapsulation efficiency is easily regulated by conditions. Passive drugs loading is to dissolve drugs in the aqueous or organic phase, and then select the appropriate method to prepare drug-containing liposomes, which is the most widely used method and suitable for the preparation of liposomes loading liposoluble drug with high affinity to phospholipid membranes.

The evaluation of liposomes mainly includes shape, particle size, surface potential, leakage rate, encapsulation efficiency, and drug loading, etc. Encapsulation efficiency is an important index for evaluating the preparation process of liposomes, which is mainly affected by the composition of membrane, aqueous phase volume, number of liposomes, and the acting force between drugs and phospholipid membranes, and drug-to-lipid ratio, etc.. This can be determined by cation exchange resin, molecular sieve, and ultrafiltration. The cation-exchange resin is used to adsorb unloaded drugs with positive charge to separate the unloaded drugs from those in the vesicles, and then the drug content is determined to calculate its encapsulation efficiency.

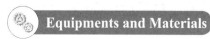 **Equipments and Materials**

1. Equipments   Flask, beaker, volumetric flask, measuring cylinder, pipette, glass wool, syringe (5ml), microinjector (100μl), microporous filter membrane (0.8μm), electronic balance, rotary evaporator, water bath, magnetic stirrer, optical microscope, ultraviolet spectrophotometer, etc.

2. Materials   Citric acid, sodium citrate, soybean phospholipid (for injection), cholesterol, ethanol, disodium hydrogen phosphate, sodium dihydrogen phosphate, berberine hydrochloride (BH), sodium bicarbonate, 732 cation exchange resin, 95% ethanol, etc.

 Experimental Methods

I. Preparation of Blank Liposomes

【Formula】

Soybean phospholipid (for injection)	1.8g
Cholesterol	0.6g
Ethanol	4ml
Citrate acid buffer	q.s.

【Procedure】

(1) Preparation of citrate acid buffer solution (pH 3.8): Weigh 10.5g of citric acid and 7.0g of sodium citrate and transfer them to a 1000ml volumetric flask, add water to dissolve and dilute to scale line, mix well, and then obtain it. Take 60ml, put it into a small beaker, and keep it warm over a water bath at 55 ~ 60℃ for later use.

(2) Weigh the formula amount of phospholipids and cholesterol and transfer them to a 100ml flask, add 4ml of ethanol, stir in a water bath at 55~60℃ to dissolve. The lipid membrane was formed on the wall of flask using a rotary evaporator to remove ethanol under reduced pressure.

(3) Add the preheated citric acid buffer solution in "(1)" into "(2)", hydrate at 55~60℃ for 10 minutes under rotation, take it out and transfer to a beaker, and stir for 20~30 minutes at room temperature on a magnetic stirrer. If the volume of solution is reduced, add distilled water to 60ml, mix well, and obtain it.

【Notes】

(1) Open flame is prohibited during the experiment.

(2) The ethanol solution of phospholipids and cholesterol should be clear and not left in the water bath for too long time.

(3) When lipid membranes are prepared, they should be as thin and uniform as possible.

(4) During hydration, it is necessary to ensure that all lipids are fully hydrated and there should be no lipid mass left on the flask wall.

II. Preparation of Passively Loaded BH Liposomes

【Formula】

Soybean phospholipid (for injection)	1.2g
Cholesterol	0.4g
Ethanol	4ml
BH solution (1mg/ml)	60ml

【Procedure】

(1) Preparation of phosphate buffer solution (PBS, pH 5.8): Weigh 0.37g of disodium hydrogen phosphate and 2.0g of sodium dihydrogen phosphate, add an appropriate amount of distilled water, dissolve and dilute to 1000ml, mix well, and then obtain it.

(2) Preparation of BH solution: Weigh a proper amount of BH and prepare a solution with a concentration of 1mg/ml by PBS (dissolved by heating over a 60℃ water bath).

(3) Weigh phospholipids and cholesterol according to the formula, transfer them into a 100ml flask, and add 4ml of ethanol. The rest of operations, except that the citrate buffer was replaced with BH solution, is according to the method under the item of "Preparation of Blank Liposomes".

III. Preparation of Remote Loaded BH Liposomes

【Formula】

Blank liposomes	2ml
Sodium bicarbonate solution	0.1ml
BH solution (3mg/ml)	1ml

【Procedure】

(1) Preparation of BH solution: Weigh an appropriate amount of BH and prepare a solution with a concentration of 3mg/ml by PBS (dissolved by heating over a 60℃ water bath).

(2) Preparation of sodium bicarbonate solution (pH 7.8): Weigh 50g of $NaHCO_3$, place it in a 1000ml volumetric flask, add water to dissolve and dilute to 1000ml, mix well, and obtain it.

(3) Remote drug loading: Transfer 2ml of blank liposome suspension (In advance, twice extrude through 0.8μm microporous membrane), 1ml of BH solution and 0.5ml of $NaHCO_3$ solution, successively add them into 10ml penicillin bottle under shaking, mix well, add plug to seal, incubate in water bath at 60℃ for 15 minutes, then immediately cool with cold water to terminate the drug loading, then obtain it.

【Notes】

(1) In the process of remote drug loading, the order of drug addition can not be reversed, and the mixture should be shaken while adding, so as to ensure even mixing and consistent gradient of each part in the system.

(2) When the water bath is kept, it is necessary to gently shake at any time (or shake by hand for 20 seconds every 1 minute), but it should ensure the uniform of the system without violent shake.

(3) It is necessary to also be shaken gently during the cooling process.

IV. Morphological Observation and Determination of Particle Size

Take the liposomes to observe their morphology under oil microscope, draw their structure, and record their maximum and minimum particle sizes. The prepared liposome liquid is passed through 0.8μm microporous filter membrane twice for pelletization, then observe the character of liposome under oil microscope, draw their structure, and record the maximum and minimum particle size of liposomes.

V. Determination of Encapsulation Efficiency

1. Preparation of cation exchange resin separation column Weigh an appropriate amount of activated cation exchange resin, suck it into a 5ml syringe with a small amount of glass wool at the bottom, add PBS to hydrate cation exchange resin, and drip dry naturally.

2. Investigation of column separation

(1) Preparation of mixture solution of BH and blank liposomes: Accurately measure out 0.1ml of BH solution (3mg/ml), place it in a small test tube, add 0.2ml of blank liposomes suspension, and mix well, then obtain it.

(2) Preparation of blank solvent: Take 6ml of ethanol (95%), place it in a 10ml volumetric flask, and add PBS to dilute to the calibration line, shake well, and obtain it.

(3) Preparation of reference solution: Accurately transfer 0.1ml of the mixture obtained at (1) into a 10ml volumetric flask, add 6ml of 95% ethanol, shake to be dissolved and clarified, add PBS to dilute to calibration line, shake well, filter, discard the initial filtrate, and transfer 4ml of the subsequent filtrate into a 10ml volumetric flask, add the blank solvent obtained in (2) to dilute to calibration line, and shake well, then obtain it.

(4) Preparation of sample solution: Accurately transfer 0.1ml of the mixture solution obtained in (1) to the top of cation exchange resin column (column length 1cm), after the top liquid disappears, place it for 5 minutes, carefully add 2~3ml of PBS (note that the resin at the top of the column not be dispersed) for elution, collect the eluate into a 10ml volumetric flask, add 6ml of 95% ethanol, shake to be dissolved and clarified, add PBS to dilute it to the calibration line, shake it to be dissolved and clear, filter and discard the initial filtrate, take the subsequent filtrate, then obtain it.

(5) Absorbance determination and calculation of column separating degree: Take blank solvent as control, determine the absorbance of sample solution and reference solution at the wavelength of 345nm, respectively, and calculate the column resolution according to the following formula.

$$\text{Column separating degree} = 1 - A_{sample}/(A_{reference} \times 2.5) \qquad (17-1)$$

Where, A_{sample} is the absorbance of sample solution, $A_{reference}$ is the absorbance of reference solution, 2.5 is the dilution ratio of reference solution to sample solution, and the column resolution value is required to be greater than 0.90.

3. Determination of entrapment efficiency Accurately pippet two samples of 0.1ml of BH liposomes, transfer one sample into a 10ml volumetric flask, operate according to the section 2(3), place the other sample on the top of the separation column, operate according to the section 2(4), determine the absorbance of the obtained solution at the wavelength of 345nm, and calculate the entrapment efficiency according to the following formula.

$$\text{Entrapment efficiency} = A_2/(A_1 \times 2.5) \times 100\% \qquad (17-2)$$

Where, A_2 is the absorbance of BH in the isolated liposomes, A_1 is the total absorbance of BH in the unisolated liposomes, and 2.5 is the dilution ratio of the unisolated liposomes to the isolated liposomes.

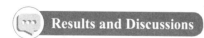 **Results and Discussions**

1. Results

(1) Take pictures of each liposome sample under the microscope and describe them.

(2) Record maximum particle size of the liposomes and the particle size of most liposomes (Table 17-1).

(3) Record the column separating degree and encapsulation efficiency (Table 17–1).

Table 17–1 Determination Results of morphology and particle size of liposomes

Liposome Sample	Description	Maximum particle size/μm	Particle size of most liposomes/μm	Column separating degree	Encapsulation efficiency/%
Blank liposome					——
BH passive loading liposome					
BH remote loading liposome					

2. Discussion

(1) Compare the advantages and disadvantages of active drug loading method with passive one in the preparation of BH liposomes and analyze their causes.

(2) Is there any differences between your experimental results and those of other groups? If yes, please analyze the reasons.

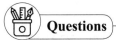 **Questions**

1. What are the main factors influencing liposome formation?

2. What are the principles and characteristics of active and passive loading of drugs into liposomes?

3. How to improve the entrapment efficiency of liposomes?

PPT

实验十八　缓释制剂的制备及释放度测定

实验目的

1. **掌握**　亲水凝胶骨架型和溶蚀性缓释片的释药机制和制备工艺。
2. **熟悉**　缓释片释放度的测定方法。

实验原理

　　缓释制剂是指在规定释放介质中，按要求缓慢地非恒速释放药物，其与相应的普通制剂比较，给药频率减少一半或有所减少，且能显著增加患者顺应性的制剂。缓释制剂药物的释放通常符合一级或 Higuchi 动力学过程。缓释制剂的设计应综合考虑药物的理化因素、机体的生物因素以及制剂的生物利用度等方面因素。

　　缓释制剂的释药原理主要基于控制溶出、扩散、扩散与溶出相结合，也可利用渗透压或离子交换机制。以扩散为主要机制的缓释给药系统中，药物先溶解形成溶液，然后再从制剂中扩散出来进入体液，其释药速率受药物扩散速率控制。扩散机制的缓控释制剂分为两类，分别是贮库型和骨架型。

　　骨架型缓释制剂是指药物和一种或多种骨架材料通过压制、融合等技术手段制成的片状、粒状或其他形式的制剂；药物以分子或结晶状态均匀分散在骨架结构中。按照所使用的骨架材料可分为亲水性凝胶骨架制剂、不溶性骨架制剂、溶蚀性骨架制剂等，其释药原理各不相同。本实验以布洛芬为模型药物，制备亲水凝胶骨架片和溶蚀性骨架片。

　　亲水凝胶骨架片（hydrophilic matrix tablet）是以亲水聚合物或天然果胶为骨架材料制备的片剂。亲水性凝胶骨架材料分为天然高分子材料类、纤维素类、非纤维素多糖、乙烯聚合物类四类；亲水性材料遇水形成凝胶层，随着凝胶层继续水化，骨架膨胀，药物可通过水凝胶层扩散释出，延缓药物的释放。

　　溶蚀性骨架片是指将药物与非水溶性可溶蚀的骨架材料混合制备的片剂，一般是通过孔道扩散与蚀解控制药物释放。溶蚀性骨架材料分为蜡类、脂肪酸及其酯类，如蜂蜡、巴西棕榈蜡、硬脂酸、硬脂醇、单硬脂酸甘油酯、氢化植物油、聚乙二醇单硬脂酸、甘油三酯等。

　　缓释制剂的质量评价一般包括制剂质量检测、体外药物释放度试验、体内试验和体内 - 体外相关性试验。体外释放度是在模拟体内消化道条件下（如温度、介质的 pH、搅拌速率等），对制剂进行药物释放速率考察的试验，是缓释制剂质量评价中必不可少的控制指标。

实验器材

1. **仪器**　单冲压片机、智能溶出仪、紫外可见分光光度仪、药筛（80 目、100 目）、分样筛（16 目、18 目）、量瓶等。
2. **材料**　布洛芬、羟丙基甲基纤维素（HPMC K10M）、乙基纤维素、乳糖、乙醇、硬脂酸镁、硬脂醇、0.4% 氢氧化钠、磷酸盐缓冲液等。

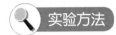 **实验方法**

（一）布洛芬亲水凝胶骨架片的制备

【处方】

布洛芬	1.5g
乙基纤维素	0.2g
羟丙基甲基纤维素 K10M	1.2g
乳糖	11.5g
硬脂酸镁	0.6g
乙醇	适量
共制得	50 片

【制法】

（1）将布洛芬、乳糖分别过 100 目筛，羟丙基甲基纤维素 K10M 过 80 目筛，混合均匀。

（2）将乙基纤维素加入乙醇制成黏合剂，加入混合粉末中制备软材，过 18 目筛制粒。

（3）将颗粒于 40~60℃ 干燥，16 目筛整粒，称重，加入硬脂酸镁混匀。

（4）计算片重，压片即得；每片含布洛芬 300mg。

【注意事项】 软材湿度要适中，否则颗粒不能成功制备；颗粒要充分干燥，否则会产生黏冲现象。

（二）布洛芬溶蚀性骨架片的制备

【处方】

布洛芬	15g
硬脂醇	1.5g
羟丙基甲基纤维素 K10M	1.2g
硬脂酸镁	0.6g
共制得	50 片

【制法】

（1）取布洛芬过 100 目筛，另将硬脂醇置于蒸发皿中，于 80℃ 水浴上加热融化，加入布洛芬搅匀，冷却，置研钵中研碎。

（2）加羟丙基甲基纤维素胶浆（以 80% 乙醇 3ml 制得）制成软材（若胶浆量不足，可再加 80% 乙醇适量），18 目筛制粒。

（3）将颗粒于 35~45℃ 干燥，16 目筛整粒，称重，加入硬脂酸镁混匀。

（4）按每片含布洛芬 300mg 计算片重，压片即得。

（三）缓释制剂释放度的考察

【标准曲线制作】 精密称取布洛芬对照品约 20mg，置于 100ml 量瓶中，用 0.4% 氢氧化钠溶液溶解，摇匀并定容。分别精密移取该溶液 2.5，5.0，7.5，10.0，12.5，15.0ml，置于 50ml 量瓶中，用 0.4% 氢氧化钠溶液定容。按分光光度法，在波长 263nm 处测定吸光度，以吸光度对浓度进行回归分析，得到标准曲线回归方程，并绘制标准曲线。

【释放度测定】 取布洛芬亲水凝胶缓释片或溶蚀型骨架缓释片，照《中国药典》2020 年版通则释放度测定法测定。

采用溶出度测定法桨法的装置，以磷酸盐缓冲液（取磷酸二氢钾 68.05g，加 1mol/L 氢氧化钠溶液 56ml，用水稀释至 10000ml，摇匀，pH 应为 6.0）900ml 为释放介质，温度为 37℃ ± 0.5℃，转速为每分钟 50 转，经 0.15，0.5，0.45，1.0，1.5，2.0，3.0，4.0，5.0，7.0，9，12 小时分别取样 10ml，同时补加同体积释放介质，样品经 0.45μm 微孔滤膜过滤，取续滤液 5ml，按照分光光度法，在 263nm 处测定吸光度。

实验结果与讨论

1. **片剂外观及质量检测** 进行片剂外观形态、平均重量、片重差异的考察，并将结果填入表 18-1。

表 18-1 布洛芬缓释片样品重量及差异

编号	1	2	3	4	5	6	7	8	9	10	11	12	13	14	15	16	17	18	19	20
亲水凝胶片重 /g																				
片重差异																				
结论																				

编号	1	2	3	4	5	6	7	8	9	10	11	12	13	14	15	16	17	18	19	20
溶蚀片片重 /g																				
片重差异																				
结论																				

亲水凝胶骨架片平均片重：＿＿＿g；溶蚀性骨架片平均片重：＿＿＿g。

2. **标准曲线的绘制** 根据表 18-2 数据绘制标准曲线。

表 18-2 布洛芬标准曲线数据

布洛芬浓度 / (mg/ml)						
吸光度（A_{263}）						

3. **累积释放率的计算和释放曲线的绘制** 根据表 18-3 数据绘制。

表 18-3 缓释片的累积释放率数据

	亲水凝胶骨架片			溶蚀性骨架片		
	1#	2#	3#	1#	2#	3#
取样时间 /h						
吸光度						
药物浓度 / (μg/ml)						
累计释放百分率 /%						

累积释放百分率按照式（18-1）计算：

$$Rel=(n×V×C)/G×100\%$$ （18-1）

式中，Rel 为累积释放百分率；n 为稀释倍数；V 为取样体积；C 为按照标准曲线计算的样品浓度；G 为缓释片平均所含布洛芬量，或标准片的标示量。

4. **讨论**

（1）比较不同处方布洛芬缓释片 1，2，4，7 小时的累计释放百分率，对释放曲线进行一级方程、Higuchi 方程、零级方程的拟合，做出评价。

（2）分析实验结果并进行讨论。

思考题

1. 口服缓释制剂的设计原则有哪些？
2. 缓释制剂的释放度实验有何意义？如何使其具有实用价值？
3. 为什么要进行制剂体外释放度与体内生物药剂学行为的相关性研究？

（陈桐楷）

Lab. 18 Preparation of the Sustained-Release Preparations and Determination of Release Rates

 Experimental Objectives

1. To master the release mechanism and preparation techniques of the hydrophilic gel and erodible matrix sustained-release tablets.

2. To familiarize with the determination methods of release rates of the sustained-release tablets.

 Experimental Principles

The sustained-release preparations are the drug formulations that releases the drug slowly and at a non constant speed according to the requirements in the specified release medium. Compared with the corresponding ordinary preparation, the dosing frequency is reduced by half or somewhat, and can improve significantly the patient's compliance. The first-order or Higuchi kinetics governs the release of sustained-preparations. The design of the formulation should take account into the necessary factors, such as physicochemical features of the drug, physiological condition, and bioavailability.

The release mechanisms of the sustained-release preparations are involved in the dissolution regulation, diffusion, or the combination of dissolution and diffusion as well as osmotic pressure or ion exchange. In the diffusion model of sustained-release preparations, the drug dissolves and diffuses into the body fluids, successively, the release rate of which is controlled by the drug diffusion rate. The diffusion mechanism of the sustainable-release preparations is categorized as reservoir and matrix type.

The matrix sustainable-release preparations in the form of tablets, granules, or other forms are referred to that the drug is evenly dispersed in the one or more matrix materials in the molecular or crystal state after compression, fusion, or other preparation process. The preparations based on the type of material used are mainly categorized as hydrophilic gel matrix, insoluble matrix, and erodible matrix preparations, involved in different release mechanisms among them. In this experiment, ibuprofen is selected as a model drug to prepare hydrophilic gel matrix tablets and erodible matrix tablets.

The drug of hydrophilic gel matrix tablets are dispersed in the hydrophilic polymer or natural pectins including natural polymers, cellulose, polysaccharides, and polyethylene polymers. The gel layer is formed when matrix contact with water, and continuously hydrates and expands, then drugs diffuse through the hydrated gel layer, which delays the drug release.

Erodible matrix tablets are the compressed tablets composed of drug and water-insoluble erodible matrix materials, and drug release is realized though the diffusion mechanisms of the formation of microchannels and degradation of matrix. Erodible matrix materials are categorized as waxes, fatty acids and their esters including beeswax, carnauba wax, stearic acid, stearyl alcohol, glyceryl monostearate, hydrogenated vegetable oil, polyethylene glycol monostearate, and triglyceride, and so on.

The quality evaluation of the sustained-release preparations contains general quality evaluation, the *in vitro* drug release rate test, the *in vivo* test, and their correlation analysis. The *in vitro* release rate serves as a crucial index of quality control of the sustained-release preparations. The *in vitro* drug release is performed in the artificially simulating of the digestive tract environment including temperature, pH and agitating rate of the media, and so forth to evaluate the release behavior of drug from tablets.

 Equipments and Materials

1. Equipments　Single-punch tablet machine, intelligent dissolution apparatus, ultraviolet-visible spectrophotometer, drug sieves (80 & 100 mesh), sample sieves (16 & 18 mesh), and volumetric flasks, etc.

2. Materials　Ibuprofen, hydroxypropyl methylcellulose (HPMC K10M), ethyl cellulose, lactose, ethanol, magnesium stearate, stearyl alcohol, 0.4% NaOH, and phosphate buffer, etc.

 Experimental Methods

Ⅰ. Preparation of Ibuprofen Hydrophilic Matrix Tablets

【Formula】

Ibuprofen	1.5g
Ethyl cellulose	0.2g
Hydroxypropyl methylcellulose K10M	1.2g
Lactose	11.5g
Magnesium stearate	0.6g
Ethanol	q.s.
Total	50 tablets

【Procedure】

(1) Sieve the ibuprofen and lactose through a 100-mesh sieve individually and hydroxypropyl methylcellulose K10M through an 80-mesh sieve, mix them evenly.

(2) Put ethyl cellulose into ethanol to prepare the adhesive, and mix with the mixed powder to prepare a soft material and sieve through an 18-mesh sieve to acquire granules.

(3) Dry the granules at 40~60℃, and sieve with a 16-mesh sieve. Weigh the dry granules and add magnesium stearate and mix properly.

(4) Calculate the tablet weight and compress tablets (300mg ibuprofen per tablet).

【Notes】To prepare the granules successfully, the humidity of soft materials should be moderate. In particular, the granules should be thoroughly dried to avoid the adhering to the punch.

Ⅱ. Preparation of Ibuprofen Erodible Matrix Tablets

【Formula】

Ibuprofen	15g
Stearyl alcohol	1.5g
Hydroxypropyl methylcellulose K10M	1.2g
Magnesium stearate	0.6g
Total	50 tablets

【Procedure】

(1) Sieve the Ibuprofen with a 100-mesh sieve. Place stearyl alcohol in an evaporating dish, heat

it melt through a water bather at 80℃, and then add the ibuprofen into it, stir and cool, last grind the mixture in a mortar.

(2) Add hydroxypropyl methylcellulose mucilage (3ml of 80% ethanol) to prepare soft material (if the mucilage amount is insufficient, add an appropriate amount of 80% ethanol again), and sieve with an 18-mesh sieve to prepare granules.

(3) Dry the granules at 35~45℃, sieve the granules with a 16-mesh sieve, weigh, add magnesium stearate, and mix evenly.

(4) Calculate the tablet weight according to 300mg ibuprofen per tablet, compress tablet.

Ⅲ. Investigating the Release Rates of the Sustained-Release Preparations

【Standard curve plot】Add 20mg of Ibuprofen reference substance in a 100ml volumetric flask, and dissolve it in the 0.4% NaOH solution, shake and make the constant volume to stock solution. In a 50ml volumetric flask, take precisely 2.5, 5.0, 7.5, 10.0, 12.5 and 15.0ml of the stock solution, and make the constant volume with 0.4% NaOH solution. Determine the absorbance at 263nm by spectrophotometry. Perform the regression analysis of the data to obtain the regression equation of the standard curve and then plot a standard curve.

【Measurement of release rate】Determine the release rate of ibuprofen hydrophilic gel or erodible matrix sustained-release tablets according to the release rate determination method mentioned in the *Chinese Pharmacopoeia*, 2020 edition.

Use the dissolution determination method with the paddle agitation to measure the release rate of ibuprofen from tablets. Add 900ml of phosphate buffer solution into release cup as the release media (68.05g of potassium dihydrogen phosphate with 56ml of 1mol/L NaOH solution, diluted to 10000ml with water, shake up and adjust its pH value to 6.0). The temperature of PBS in the cup is set at 37℃±0.5℃, with a rotating speed of 50r/min. Then, collect 10ml of release media at 0.15, 0.5, 0.45, 1.0, 1.5, 2.0, 3.0, 4.0, 5.0, 7.0, 9 and 12h after begin agitation, simultaneously add the same volume of the release media. The samples are filtered through 0.45μm microporous filter membranes. The absorbance of the continuous filtrate (5ml) is determined at 263nm by spectrophotometry.

Results and Discussions

1. Appearance and quality evaluation of tablets The appearance, average weight, and the weight variation of the tablets are investigated, and the results are recorded in the Table 18-1.

Table 18−1　Sample weight and difference of Ibuprofen sustained-release tablets

No.	1	2	3	4	5	6	7	8	9	10	11	12	13	14	15	16	17	18	19	20
Hydrophilic gel tablet weight/g																				
Tablet weight variation																				
Conclusion																				
No.	1	2	3	4	5	6	7	8	9	10	11	12	13	14	15	16	17	18	19	20
Erodible matrix tablet tablet weight/g																				
Tablet weight variation																				
Conclusion																				

Hydrophilic gel matrix tablet average tablet weight: _____g; erodible matrix tablet average tablet weight: _____g.

2. The drawing of the standard curve (Table 18-2)

Table 18-2   The standard curve of ibuprofen

Ibuprofen concentration/(mg/ml)						
Absorbance (A_{263})						

3. Calculation of the accumulated release rate and plot of the release curve (Table 18-3)

Table 18-3   The accumulated release rate of the sustained-release tablets

	Hydrophilic gel matrix tablets			Erodible matrix tablets		
	1#	2#	3#	1#	2#	3#
Sampling time/h						
Absorbance						
Drug concentration/(μg/ml)						
Accumulated release percentage/%						

The accumulated release percentage can be calculated by the following formula:

$$Rel=(n \times V \times C)/G \times 100\% \tag{18-1}$$

Where, *Rel* is the accumulated release percentage; *n* is the dilution multiples; *V* is the sampling volume; *C* is the sample concentration based on the standard curve; *G* is the average content of the ibuprofen in the sustained-release tablets or labeled amount of the standard tablet.

4. Discussions

(1) Compare the accumulated release percentage of the ibuprofen sustained-release tablets with different prescription after 1, 2, 4, 7h release, and fit the release curve via a first-order equation, Higuchi equation, and zero-order equation. Evaluate the different outcomes of all tablets.

(2)   Analyze the experimental results and discuss the outcomes.

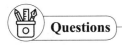 **Questions**

1. What are the design principles of oral sustained-release preparations?

2. What is the significance of the release test of the sustained-release preparations? How to make it practical?

3. What is the purpose of correlation studies of the *in vitro* release rate of preparations and the *in vivo* biopharmaceutical behaviors?

实验十九　药物制剂的稳定性实验

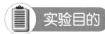 **实验目的**

1. **掌握**　应用经典恒温实验法预测制剂有效期的方法。
2. **熟悉**　制剂稳定性考察项目和方法。

实验原理

药物制剂的稳定性系指药物制剂在生产、运输、贮藏、销售直至临床应用前的一系列过程中质量变化的速度和程度。稳定性是评价药物制剂质量的重要指标之一，也是核定药物制剂使用期限的主要依据。药物制剂的稳定性一般涉及化学、物理、生物学三个方面。

稳定性实验方法主要有影响因素法、长期试验法（留样观察法）、加速试验法、经典恒温法等。影响因素法一般常用于原料药、制剂处方和工艺设计，而药物制剂有效期的预测多采用长期试验法和加速实验法，经典恒温法不能用于新药研究，但可用于溶液型药物制剂的稳定性研究或有效期预测，为制定有效期提供参考。

经典恒温法的理论依据是 Arrhenius 指数定律：$K = Ae^{\frac{-E}{RT}}$，其对数形式即

$$\lg K = -\frac{E}{2.303\ RT} + \lg A \qquad (19\text{-}1)$$

式中，K 为反应速度常数；T 为绝对温度；$\lg K$ 与 $1/T$ 呈线性。

在一定温度下，药物降解过程多为一级或伪一级反应。一级反应药物浓度与时间的关系式为

$$\lg C = -\frac{Kt}{2.303} + \lg C_0 \qquad (19\text{-}2)$$

式中，C_0 为初始浓度；t 为反应时间；C 为 t 时反应物的浓度。

通常将药物在室温（25℃）下降解10%所需的时间（$t_{0.9}$）作为有效期，当药物降解是一级反应时，计算公式为

$$t_{0.9} = \frac{0.1054}{K} \qquad (19\text{-}3)$$

一级反应的有效期与制剂中药物的初浓度无关，而与速度常数 K 值成反比。

经典恒温法的实验步骤：①预实验。确定指标性成分并建立分析方法，初步了解药物稳定性情况；通常选择药物不稳定的活性成分或指标成分作为考核指标，测定方法应灵敏、准确，能反应加速试验过程中指标成分的浓度（含量）变化，进而反映药物的稳定性。②实验设计。选定实验条件、设计实验温度（4个以上不同温度）和取样时间点（5个以上时间点）。③确定反应级数。在不同温度下进行实验，分别于不同时间点取样，测定药物浓度，以 $\lg C$ 对 t 作图，得一条直线，则为一级反应。④求 $K_{25℃}$。根据不同温度的 $\lg C$ 对 t 图，计算不同温度反应速度常数 K。再以 $\lg K$ 对 $1/T$ 作图，将直线外推到25℃，求出 $K_{25℃}$。⑤根据公式（19-3）计算有

效期 $t_{0.9}$。

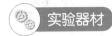

实验器材

1. **仪器**　超级恒温水浴、碘量瓶（150ml）、移液管（1、2、5、10ml）、酸式滴定管、洗瓶等。

2. **材料**　维生素 C 注射剂、碘液（$0.1mol \cdot L^{-1}$）、稀醋酸、淀粉指示剂等。

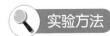

实验方法

（一）含量测定方法

精密量取维生素 C 注射液 2ml 置于碘量瓶中，加蒸馏水 15ml、丙酮 2ml，摇匀，放置 5 分钟，加稀醋酸 4ml，淀粉指示液 1ml，用 $0.1mol \cdot L^{-1}$ 碘液滴定，至溶液呈蓝色并持续 30 秒钟不褪，记录消耗碘液的毫升数（每毫升碘液相当于维生素 C 8.806mg）。

（二）经典恒温试验

将同一批号的维生素 C 注射液样品分别置于 4 个不同温度的超级恒温水浴中，温度和取样时间见表 19-1。当水浴温度至设置温度时，即投入维生素 C 注射液，待药液与水浴温度相等时，即取出立即冷却，并按（一）法进行含量测定，作为起始浓度 C_0，剩余安瓿继续恒温放置至规定时间，取出立即冷却，并测定剩余维生素 C 的含量，记作 C_n。

（三）实验数据处理

（1）记录含量测定时消耗碘液的毫升数，以不同温度下未经加热的样品所消耗碘液的毫升数（即初始浓度 V_0）为 100% 相对浓度，各温度下经加热样品所消耗碘液的毫升数（V_n）与初始浓度相比，计算各自的相对浓度，即 $C_n = (V_n / V_0) \times C_0 \times 100\%$，数据记录于表 19-1 中。

（2）由公式（19-1）计算各实验温度下维生素 C 降解的速度常数 K。将各试验温度下，不同降解时间为横坐标（$X \to t$），对应的样品相对百分浓度的对数为纵坐标（$Y \to lgC$）进行回归，计算各实验温度下的回归方程、相关系数，推导各温度的降解速度常数 K。

（3）计算室温（25℃）时维生素 C 降解速度常数 $K_{25℃}$。由式（19-2）可求得 $K_{25℃}$，或将 $lgk \to 1/T$ 作图，由图中的直线外延至室温求得。

（4）计算室温时的 $t_{0.9}$。由式（19-3）可求得室温 25℃时分解 10% 需要的时间。

实验结果与讨论

1. **结果**　实验安排及测定数据见表 19-1 所示，实验数据处理结果见表 19-2 所示。

表 19-1　实验安排

温度 T/K	取样时间 /h	消耗碘液数 /ml	相对浓度 $C/\%$	浓度对数 lgC	回归结果
333	0				
	24				
	48				
	72				
	96				
	120				

续表

温度 T/K	取样时间 /h	消耗碘液数 /ml	相对浓度 C/%	浓度对数 $\lg C$	回归结果
343	0				
	12				
	24				
	36				
	48				
	60				
353	0				
	6				
	12				
	18				
	24				
	30				
363	0				
	3				
	6				
	9				
	12				
	15				

表 19-2　数据处理结果

试验温度 T/K	取样时间点 /h	速度常数 K/h^{-1}	$\lg k$	$K_{25℃}$/h^{-1}	$t_{0.9}$/h
333	24				
343	12				
353	6				
363	3				

2. 讨论

（1）碘量法测定维生素 C 含量时，加入稀醋酸、丙酮的目的是什么？

（2）加速实验时，取出注射剂为何需立即冷却？

（3）分析影响实验结果准确性的因素和关键操作。

思考题

1. 试分析中药复方制剂与化学药物制剂稳定性研究有何差异。

2. 通过影响维生素 C 氧化的因素，讨论防止药物氧化的措施有哪些。

3. 如果药物制剂需低温贮存，应该怎样制定其稳定性研究方案？

（郑　琴）

Lab. 19 The Stability Experiment of Pharmaceutical Preparation

Experimental Objectives

1. To master the method of predicting the stability of pharmaceutical preparation by applying the classical thermostatic method.

2. To be familiar with items and methods of preparation stability inspection.

Experimental Principles

The stability of pharmaceutical preparation refers to the speed and degree of quality changes in a series of processes such as manufacture, transportation, storage, sale till to clinical application. Stability is one of the important indicators to evaluate the quality of pharmaceutical preparations, and it is also the main basis for verifying shelf life of pharmaceutical preparations. Stability generally involves three aspects: chemistry, physics and biology.

The methods for stability experiment mainly include the influence factor method, the long-term test method (reserving sample observation method), the accelerated test method, the classical thermostatic method and so on. The influence factor method is generally used in researches of the stability of raw materials, prescription and compounding process design. Long-term test and accelerated test methods are often used in shelf life estimation of pharmaceutical product. However, the classical thermostatic method can not be used for new drug research, it can only be used in researches on the stability or validity prediction of solution-type preparation, which provides reference for the effective period of preparation.

The theory of classical thermostatic method is based on the Arrhenius Exponential law. The mathematical expression is $K=Ae^{\frac{-E}{RT}}$, and the log form is

$$\lg K=-\frac{E}{2.303\,RT}+\lg A \tag{19-1}$$

Where, K is the specific reaction rate constant and T is absolute temperature.

From the equation, $\lg K$ is linear with $1/T$. Most commonly, first-order or pseudo-first-order rate reactions are encountered in pharmacy at a certain temperature. In the first-order reaction, the relationship between drug concentration and time can be described as mathematical expression

$$\lg C=-\frac{Kt}{2.303}+\lg C_0 \tag{19-2}$$

Where, C_0 is the initial concentration of the drug, t is the reaction time, C is the concentration of intact drug remaining.

Shelf life ($t_{0.9}$) is the time required for the drug to degrade with 90% of the intact drug remaining at room temperature (25℃).The shelf-life equation for a first-order reaction is

$$t_{0.9} = \frac{0.1054}{K} \tag{19-3}$$

From the equation, the shelf-life is not related to the initial concentration of the drug, but is inversely proportional with the specific reaction rate constant.

The experimental procedure of classical thermostatic method are as follows:

1. Pre-experiment: Select some components or active ingredients, normally unstable, as indicator ingredients in the experiment and establish the analytical methods. It should be sensitive, accurate, which can reflect the concentration (content) of the indicator ingredients' changes in the acceleration experiment, and thus reflect the stability of the drug.

2. Experiment Design: Select experimental conditions and set 4 or more different experimental temperatures, and 5 or more sampling time points.

3. Determination of the reaction order: Carried out the experiments at different temperatures, sample at different time points and determine to ascertain the rate order of reactions. If $\lg C$ is linear with t, the reaction is a first-order rate.

4. Calculation of $K_{25℃}$: Draw $\lg C$-t plot of different temperatures and make a linear fit, calculate the specific reaction rate constant (K) under different temperatures from the slope, draw $\lg K$-$1/T$ plot and make a linear fit, then extrapolate the line to the temperature 25℃ and calculate $K_{25℃}$.

5. Calculate shelf life ($t_{0.9}$) by the equation 19-3.

 Equipments and Materials

1. Equipments　Thermostatic water bath, iodine flask (150ml), pipette (1ml, 2ml, 5ml, 10ml), acid burette, washing bottle, etc.

2. Materials　Vitamin C injections, iodine solution (0.1mol · L⁻¹), diluted acetic acid, starch indicator, etc.

 Experimental Methods

I. Content Determination Method

Measure accurately 2ml of vitamin C injection in a iodine flask, add 15ml of distilled water, 2ml of acetone, shake well, and maintain for 5 minutes. After that, add 4ml of dilute acetic acid, 1ml of starch indicator solution, titrate with 0.1mol · L⁻¹ iodine solution until the solution turns blue and does not fade for 30 seconds, record the number of milliliters of iodine solution consumed (each milliliter of iodine solution is equivalent to 8.806mg of vitamin C).

II. Classic Thermostatic Test

The same batch of vitamin C injection ampoule will be put into four different thermostatic water baths (in four different set temperatures) when the temperature reach to that is set. The detail of temperature and sampling time are shown in the Table 19-1. After a while, when the temperature inside the ampoule is the same as the bath, several ampoule will be take out of the bath to be determined according to content measurement method 1 to get the content of vitamin C as original concentration C_0 in different temperatures. The remain ampoule will be placed for different time, and being sampled (immediately cooling) following the table and determined the content of vitamin C in ampoule (recorded as C_n).

III. Data Analysis

(1) The volume (V_0) of iodine solution consumed by vitamin C injection unheated in different temperatures is recorded as 100% relative concentration. The volume (V_n) of iodine solution consumed by vitamin C injection heated in different temperature for different times are recorded. The ratio of V_n to V_0 are recorded as relative concentration (C_n) in different temperatures at different times. The equation is $C_n = (V_n / V_0) \times C_0 \times 100\%$. All the data will be filled in the Table 19–1.

(2) Calculate specific reaction rate constant K according to the equation 19-1. The different degradation time is X-axis ($X \rightarrow t$)and the corresponding logarithm of relative concentration is Y-axis ($Y \rightarrow \lg C$). Draw $\lg C$- t plot of different temperatures and make a linear fit, then calculate the specific reaction rate constant (K) under different temperatures from the slope.

(3) Draw $\lg K$- $1/T$ plot and make a linear fit, then extrapolate the line to the temperature 25℃ and calculate $K_{25℃}$ according the following equation 19-2.

(4) Calculate shelf life ($t_{0.9}$) by the equation 19-3. That is the time required for a drug to decrease by 10% of original concentration at room temperature (25℃).

Results and Discussion

1. Results　The experimental arrangement and measurement data are shown in the Table 19–1. The calculation results can be filled in the Table 19–2.

Table 19–1　Experimental arrangements and measurement data

Test temperature T/K	Sampling time point/h	Volume of iodine consumed/ml	Relative concentration C/%	Logarithm of Concentration $\lg C$	Regression Equation and Correlation Factor r
333	0				
	24				
	48				
	72				
	96				
	120				
343	0				
	12				
	24				
	36				
	48				
	60				
353	0				
	6				
	12				
	18				
	24				
	30				

Continued

Test temperature T/K	Sampling time point/h	Volume of iodine consumed/ml	Relative concentration C/%	Logarithm of Concentration $\lg C$	Regression Equation and Correlation Factor r
363	0				
	3				
	6				
	9				
	12				
	15				

Table 19-2　Calculation Results

Test temperature T/K	Sampling time point/h	Speed constant K/h^{-1}	$\lg K$	$K_{25℃}$/h^{-1}	$t_{0.9}$/h
333					
343					
353					
363					

2. Discussions

(1) Analyze and discuss the purpose of adding diluted acetic acid and acetone in determination the content of vitamin C by iodimetry.

(2) Analyze and discuss the reason why the injection ampoule should be cooled immediately after taken out of the bath in the experiment.

(3) Analyze the results and discuss the key factors and operations influencing on the accuracy of the results.

 Questions

1. What are the differences in stability researches between Chinese medicine compound formulation and chemical drug preparation?

2. What are the measures to prevent the oxidation of vitamin C through factors that affecting on oxidation of vitamin C?

3. If a pharmaceutical preparation needs to be stored at low temperature, how should we formulate its stability research program?

实验二十 设计性试验

实验目的

1. **掌握** 药物制剂处方前研究的方法与内容。
2. **熟悉** 根据药物性质和治疗需要等要求，进行药物剂型设计的思路。
3. **了解** 注射剂与胶囊剂处方工艺筛选、质量评价的研究内容与方法。

实验指导

（一）化学药物：维生素 C 注射剂

常用于防治坏血病、促进创伤及骨折愈合等。维生素 C 在干燥状态下较稳定，但在潮湿状态或溶液中其分子结构中的烯二醇式结构被很快氧化，生成黄色双酮化合物。虽仍有药效，但会迅速进一步氧化、断裂，生成一系列有色的无效物质。维生素 C 对氧气、pH、金属离子、温度较为敏感。因此，为使注射剂安全、稳定、有效，在制备时必须控制温度、调节 pH 以及加入金属离子络合剂、抗氧剂等附加剂。

（二）中药：双黄连胶囊

本品由黄芩、金银花、连翘组成，用于外感风热所致的感冒，症见发热、咳嗽、咽痛。黄芩主要含有黄芩苷、黄芩素等成分。金银花主要含有绿原酸、木犀草素等成分。连翘主要含有连翘酯苷、连翘苷等成分。本方日服剂量较大，故应对药材进行提取分离精制后，再制备成各种剂型。硬胶囊制备时，需根据内容物的粉体学特性、服用剂量，来筛选辅料、空胶囊大小（囊号），再进行胶囊的填充。

实验器材

1. **仪器** 托盘天平、水浴锅、电磁炉 / 电炉、熔封仪、热压灭菌器、澄明度检查台、崩解仪、烘箱、手工胶囊填充板、乳钵、药筛、不锈钢托盘、精密 pH 试纸、纸浆、微孔滤膜、明胶空心胶囊、烧杯（1000ml）、量筒（100ml）、垂熔玻璃漏斗、安瓿（2ml）、注射器等。

2. **材料** 维生素 C、金银花饮片、黄芩饮片、连翘饮片等。

实验方法

（一）维生素 C 注射剂

1. **文献研究** 查阅相关文献，总结维生素 C 的性质特点、临床应用，提出维生素 C 注射剂的设计思路；总结注射剂的常用辅料、处方筛选、制备工艺流程和质量评价方法。

（1）药物特点与临床应用

（2）维生素 C 注射剂设计理由

（3）常用辅料及用量（表 20-1）

表 20-1　常用辅料及用量

序号	添加剂种类	附加剂	浓度范围 /%
1	抗氧剂	焦亚硫酸钠 亚硫酸氢钠 亚硫酸钠 硫代硫酸钠	0.1~0.2 0.1~0.2 0.1~0.2 0.1
2			
3			
4			
5			
6			
……			

（4）制备方法与流程

（5）质量评价项目（表 20-3）

2. 处方设计与分析（表 20-2）

表 20-2　维生素 C 注射剂处方设计与分析

序号	主药 / 添加剂	作用	用量	选择依据
1	维生素 C	主药		
2				
3				
4				
5				

备注：维生素 C 在注射剂中浓度为 5%。

3. 制备工艺

（1）注射用水的制备

① 注射用水的制备流程

② 注射用水的质量标准

（2）容器与处理

① 容器的种类

② 容器的处理

（3）维生素 C 注射剂的制备

① 药液的配制

② 过滤与灌封

③ 灭菌与检漏

4. 质量控制（表 20-3）

表 20-3 维生素 C 注射剂质量控制项目检查记录表

序号	检查项目	方法	结果
1			
2			
3			
4			
5			
......			

5. 实验结果与讨论

（1）结果　对实验结果进行叙述，并对实验得到的样品进行自我评价。画出维生素 C 注射剂的制备工艺流程图。

（2）讨论　对剂型设计、处方筛选、制备工艺中存在的问题和注意事项进行分析。

（二）双黄连胶囊

1. 文献研究　查阅相关文献，总结双黄连处方各药味的有效成分性质特点，提出该药物处方的提取工艺流程、剂型的设计思路和质量评价方法；查阅硬胶囊剂常用辅料、处方筛选、制备方法与流程和质量评价方法。

（1）药物的有效成分、提取分离和质量评价方法

（2）双黄连硬胶囊剂型设计理由

（3）常用辅料及用量（表 20-4）

表 20-4 常用辅料及用量

序号	附加剂种类	附加剂名称	用量范围 /%
1	填充剂	淀粉 糊精	
2	黏合剂		
3			
4			
5			
......			

（4）制备方法与工艺流程

（5）质量评价项目（表 20-6）

2. 处方设计与分析（表20-5）

表20-5　双黄连胶囊处方设计

序号	主药/添加剂	作用	用量	选择依据
1	黄芩、金银花、连翘	主药		
2				
3				
4				
……				

3. 制备工艺

（1）药材饮片的提取　考察比较提取方法、提取时间、溶剂及其用量。

（2）提取液的分离纯化方法

（3）辅料和处方的筛选

（4）内容物的制备

（5）胶囊剂的制备

① 胶囊壳囊号的选择

② 药物的填充

③ 硬胶囊的抛光

（6）制备方法与流程

4. 质量控制（表20-6）

表20-6　双黄连胶囊质量控制项目

序号	检查项目	方法	结果
1			
2			
3			
4			
5			
……			

5. 实验结果与讨论

（1）结果　对实验结果进行叙述，并对实验得到的样品进行自我评价，并画出实验流程图。

（2）讨论　对双黄连胶囊中药材饮片的提取分离、剂型设计、处方筛选、制备工艺中存在的问题和注意事项进行分析。

思考题

1. 药物剂型选择的依据是什么？

2. 阐述药物剂型对药物"安全、有效、稳定、可控"的影响作用。

3. 对比中药与化学药物剂型设计思路的异同。

（郑　琴）

Lab. 20 | Design Experiments

 Experimental Objectives

1. To master the research methods and contents in pre-formulation studies of pharmaceutical preparations.

2. To be familiar with the general considerations in dosage form design according to the drug properties and treatment needs.

3. To understand with the contents and methods of the formulation screening and quality evaluation of injection and capsule prescription.

 Experimental Introduction

I. Chemical Medicine: Vitamin C Injection

Vitamin C injection is generally used for the prevention and treatment of scurvy, the promotion of trauma and fracture healing, etc. Vitamin C is stable in a dry state, however, in wet situation or solution its molecular structure of the enediol structure will be quickly oxidized and thus produces yellow diketone compound. Although it still remain efficacy after that, it will be quickly followed with further oxidation, fracture and form a series of ineffective substances with color. Vitamin C is sensitive with oxygen, pH, metal ions, temperature, so it is necessary to control the temperature, adjust pH, add metal ion complexagent, antioxidant and other additives in preparation of injection in order to ensure it safety, stability and effectiveness.

II. Traditional Chinese Medicine: Shuanghuanglian Capsule

Shuanghuanglian capsule, composed of scutellaria, honeysuckle and forsythia, general used to treat colds caused by external sensation of wind fever with symptom of fever, cough, sore throat. The main components of scutellaria are baicalin, baicalein, etc. The main components honeysuckle of are chlorogenic acid, luteolin, etc. The main components of forsythia are forsythiaside and forsythin, etc. Because of a large dose, the herbs needed to be extracted, separated and refined before they are made into a dosage forms of various types. It is necessary to select proper excipients for developing the formulation and select the capsule size according to the powder properties of the contents and daily dose before we filling the empty hard gelatin capsules shells to prepare capsule dosage form.

 Equipments and Materials

1. Equipments Table balance, water bath, electromagnetic furnace/electric furnace, melting sealing instrument, pressure sterilizer, transpareance inspection machine, disintegration tester, bake out furnace, handoperated capsule-filling machine, mortar, pharmacopoeia sieve, stainless steel trays,

149

accurate range pH test paper, paper pulp, millipore filters, gelatin empty capsules, beaker (1000ml), measuring cylinder (100ml), sintered glass funnel, ampoule (2ml), syringe, etc.

2. Materials Vitamin C, decoction pieces of scutellaria, honeysuckle and forsythia, etc.

 Experimental Methods

I. Vitamin C Injection

1. Document research Review the relevant documents and summarize the characteristic features, clinical use of vitamin C, put forward the idea of dosage form design for vitamin C injection. Summarize the frequently-used excipients, prescription developing method and technological process and quality control for preparation injections.

(1) Drug characteristics and clinical use

(2) The idea of dosage form design for vitamin C injection

(3) Frequently-used excipients and usage (Table 20–1)

Table 20–1 Frequently-used excipients and usage

Serial number	Types of excipients	Excipients	Usage range /%
1	Antioxidant	Sodium pyrosulfite Sodium hydrogen sulfite Sodium sulfite Sodium thiosulfate	0.1~0.2 0.1~0.2 0.1~0.2 0.1
2			
3			
4			
5			
6			
……			

(4) Technological process and methods for preparation injections

(5) Quality control items (Table 20–3)

2. Formulation design and analysis (Table 20–2)

Table 20–2 Vitamin C injection formula and analysis

Serial number	Main drug/excipients	Role	Amount	Select reason
1	Vitamin C	Main medicine		
2				
3				
4				
5				

Note: Vitamin C is 5% in injections.

3. Procedure

(1) Preparation of water for injection

① Preparation process of water for injection

② Quality standards for water for injection

(2) Containers and treatment

① Types of containers

② Treatments of containers

(3) Preparation of VC injections

① Preparation of solution

② Filtration and sealing

③ Sterilization and leak detection

4. Quality control (Table 20–3)

Table 20–3   Vitamin C injection quality control items checklist

Serial number	Items	Methods	Results
1			
2			
3			
4			
5			
……			

5. Results and discussions

(1) Results   Describe the results of the experiment and give a self evaluation on the samples prepared in the experiment. Draw out the preparation flow-process diagram of vitamin C injection.

(2) Discussions   Analyze and discuss on problems and points for attention in the dosage form design, prescription developing and preparation process.

II. Shuanghuanglian Capsule

1. Document Research   Review the relevant documents and summarize the characteristic features of ingredients in the herbal drug in Shuanghuanglian prescription, put forward the idea of extraction process, dosage form design and quality control method. Summarize the frequently used excipients, prescription developing method and technological process and quality control for hard capsule dosage form.

(1) Characteristic features of ingredients, extraction and separation process and quality control method

(2) The idea of dosage form design for Shuanghuanglian hard capsule

(3) Frequently-used excipients and usage (Table 20–4)

Table 20−4 Frequently-used excipients and usage

Serial number	Types of excipients	Excipients	Usage range/%
1	Fillers	Starch Dextrin	
2	Binders		
3			
4			
5			
......			

(4) Technological process and methods for preparation capsules

(5) Quality control items (Table 20−6)

2. Formulation design and analysis (Table 20−5)

Table 20−5 Shuanghuanglian capsule formula and analysis

Serial number	Main drug/excipients	Role	Amount	Select reason
1	Scutellaria, Honeysuckle Forsythia	Main medicine		
2				
3				
4				
......				

3. Procedure

(1) Extraction of decoction pieces of the herbs

Research and compare extraction methods, extraction time, solvents and their amount.

(2) Separation and purification method

(3) Screening of excipients and develop a prescription

(4) Preparation of contents in capsules

(5) Preparation of capsule dosage form

① Selection of the size of capsule empty shells

② Filling of the drug

③ Polishing of the hard capsule

(6) Preparation methods and processes

4. Quality control (Table 20−6)

Table 20−6 Shuanghuanglian quality control item checklist

Serial number	Items	Methods	Results
1			
2			
3			
4			
5			
......			

5. Results and discussions

(1) Results   Describe the results of the experiment and give a self evaluation on the samples prepared in the experiment. Draw out the preparation flow-process diagram of Shuanghuanglian Capsule.

(2) Discussions   Analyze and discuss on problems and points for attention in the extraction and separation of decoctions in Shuanghuanglian capsule prescription and the dosage form design, prescription developing, preparation process.

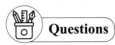 **Questions**

1. What is the basis for drug dosage form design?

2. State the influence factors of dosage form on the safety, effectiveness, stability and controllability of medicines.

3. Compare the similarities and differences between Chinese medicine and chemical medicine in dosage form design.

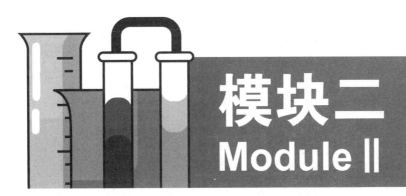

模块二
Module II

制剂评价技术
Evaluation Technologies of Pharmaceutical Preparations

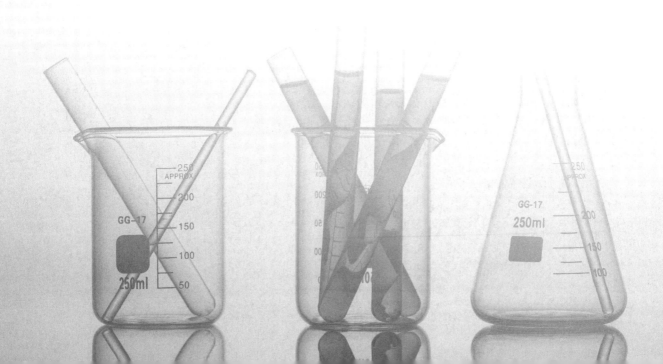

实验二十一 药物溶解度与油水分配系数的测定

 实验目的

1. **掌握** 药物溶解度与油水分配系数的测定方法。
2. **熟悉** 影响药物溶解度与油水分配系数的因素。

实验原理

药物的溶解度与油水分配系数是制剂处方前研究的主要内容，是药物剂型设计的重要依据，其性质显著影响药物的吸收和体内生物利用度。

药物的溶解度是指在一定温度（气体在一定压力）下，在定量溶剂中达到溶解平衡时（形成饱和溶液）所溶解的最大药量，通常采用在一定温度下100g溶剂中溶解溶质的最大克数来表示。根据药物在溶剂中是否发生解离或缔合，溶解度分为特性溶解度和表观溶解度。如药物在溶剂中不发生解离、缔合或其他相互作用，此时溶解度称为特性溶解度，反之则称为表观溶解度。影响药物溶解度的因素主要有药物的晶型、粒径、温度、pH、离子强度及其他添加物，在测定过程中应充分考虑上述因素的影响。

油水分配系数是指在一定温度下，药物在互不相溶的两相溶剂中分配达到平衡时，药物在两相中浓度的比值，用于表示药物分子的亲水性或亲油性的倾向，与药物的吸收密切相关。由于正辛醇的溶解度参数和细胞类脂膜的溶解度参数最为接近，因此，在制剂研究中常采用正辛醇 – 水分配系数来表示药物的油水分配系数。油水分配系数（p）计算公式：

$$p = \frac{C_o}{C_w} = \frac{(C - C_w)}{C_w} \tag{21-1}$$

式中，C_o 为平衡时药物在油相中的浓度；C_w 为平衡时药物在水相中的浓度；C 为最初水相（待分配水溶液）的药物浓度。

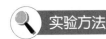 **实验器材**

1. **仪器** 锥形瓶、碘瓶、微孔滤膜、烧杯、移液管、容量瓶、磁力搅拌器、紫外 – 可见分光光度计等。
2. **材料** 氟尿嘧啶、正辛醇、蒸馏水等。

实验方法

（一）氟尿嘧啶溶解度测定

1. **药物溶解平衡时间的确定** 称取氟尿嘧啶约1g，放入碘瓶中，加水50ml，置于磁力搅拌器上进行搅拌溶解。分别于15、30、45、60、75、90、105、120、135、150分钟时以注射器吸取该溶液约 3ml，微孔滤膜（0.45μm）滤过，取续滤液 0.1ml 于 100ml 容量瓶中，加水稀释至刻度，混合均匀后于 265nm 处测定其吸光度，当相邻两个时间点的溶液吸光度差值小于 ±0.004 时所对应的时间为溶解平衡时间。

2. 药物饱和溶液浓度的测定　取上述平衡时间点的溶液样品三份，分别经微孔滤膜过滤，取续滤液 0.1ml 于 100ml 容量瓶中，加水稀释至刻度，混匀后于 265nm 处测定其吸光度，根据吸收系数（$E_{1cm}^{1\%}$）522，计算其浓度，即为氟尿嘧啶的溶解度。

（二）氟尿嘧啶在正辛醇 / 水中分配系数的测定

1. 氟尿嘧啶浓度计算　称取氟尿嘧啶约 0.5g，精密称定，放入碘瓶中，加水 100ml，摇匀，静置 1 小时，吸取该溶液约 20ml，微孔滤膜滤过，弃去初滤液，续滤液置于小烧杯中，此溶液为母液。吸取母液 0.1ml 于 100ml 容量瓶中，加水稀释至刻度，混合均匀后于 265nm 处测定其吸光度，根据吸收系数（$E_{1cm}^{1\%}$）522，计算氟尿嘧啶的浓度 C。

2. 氟尿嘧啶水溶液浓度计算　取上述母液 10ml 置于碘瓶中，加入正辛醇 10ml，置磁力搅拌器上搅拌 1 小时，静置分层。用移液管精密吸取碘瓶底部溶液 0.1ml，置于 100ml 容量瓶中，加水稀释至刻度，混合均匀后于 265nm 处测定其吸光度，根据吸收系数（$E_{1cm}^{1\%}$）522，计算氟尿嘧啶水溶液的浓度 C_w。

💬 实验结果与讨论

1. 氟尿嘧啶在水中溶解度测定结果

（1）将不同时间氟尿嘧啶溶液的吸光度记录于表 21-1。

表 21-1　不同时间氟尿嘧啶溶液的吸光度

时间 /min	15	30	45	60	75	90	105	120	135	150
吸光度（A）										

根据表中吸光度数值确定平衡时间为_____。

（2）氟尿嘧啶的溶解度结果记录于表 21-2。

表 21-2　氟尿嘧啶在水中的溶解度

编号	1	2	3	平均值
吸光度（A）				
浓度 /（g/100ml）				

2. 氟尿嘧啶在正辛醇 / 水中分配系数的测定结果

（1）将氟尿嘧啶在水溶液中的吸光度记录于表 21-3，计算其平均浓度。

表 21-3　氟尿嘧啶水溶液的吸光度和浓度

编号	1	2	3	平均值
吸光度（A）				
浓度（C）				

（2）氟尿嘧啶在正辛醇 / 水中分配平衡后水溶液的吸光度记录于表 21-4，计算其平均浓度。

表 21-4 氟尿嘧啶在正辛醇 / 水中分配平衡后水溶液的吸光度和浓度

编号	1	2	3	平均值
吸光度（A）				
浓度（C_w）				

（3）分配系数的计算。根据上述 C 和 C_w 的平均值，计算氟尿嘧啶的正辛醇 / 水分配系数。

3. 讨论

（1）本实验测定的药物溶解度为何种溶解度，为什么？

（2）实验过程中温度的控制对结果有何影响？

（3）与其他实验小组结果进行对比，是否存在差异？请分析原因。

思考题

1. 影响药物溶解度的因素主要有哪些？

2. 药物的特性溶解度与表观溶解度有何不同？

3. 油水分配系数在制剂设计中有何用途？

（陈桐楷）

Lab. 21 Measurement of Drug Solubility and Oil-Water Partition Coefficient

 Experimental Objectives

1. To master the measuring methods of solubility and oil-water partition coefficient of the drugs.
2. To be familiar with the factors affecting the solubility and oil-water partition coefficient of drugs.

 Experimental Principles

The solubility and oil-water partition coefficient of drugs are the main content of pre formulation research, and are the important basis of dosage form design, which significantly affect the absorption and bioavailability of drugs *in vivo*.

The drug solubility refers to the maximum amount of a solute in the solvent, when the dissolution equilibrium occurs to form saturated solution, at a given temperature (gas under an absolute pressure). Generally, solubility is expressed as the maximum grams of solute dissolved in 100g solvent at a given temperature. The solubility of the drug can be categorized as an intrinsic or apparent solubility, based on whether the drug dissociates, associates, or other interactions in the solvent. In the case of an intrinsic solubility, the drug does not show the dissociation, association, or any other interaction with the solvent; contrarily, it is an apparent solubility. The foremost factors that influence the drug solubility are crystal form of drug, particle size, temperature, pH value, ionic strength, and additives, which are fully considered during measurements.

The oil/water partition coefficient refers to the ratio of drug concentration in two immiscible phases, when the drug distribution in immiscible two-phase solvent approaches equilibrium at a given temperature. It indicates the hydrophilic or lipophilic tendency of the drug molecules, which closely related to the drug absorption. Because the solubility parameter of the octanol is closest to that of cell lipid membrane, the oil/water partition coefficients of drugs are usually reflected by the octanol/water partition coefficient (P), which can be calculated by the following formula:

$$p=\frac{C_o}{C_w}=\frac{(C-C_w)}{C_w} \tag{21-1}$$

Where, C_o is the concentration of drug in the oil phase at equilibrium, C_w is the concentration of drug in the water phase at equilibrium, C is the initial drug concentration in the water phase.

 Equipments and Materials

1. Equipments Conical flasks, iodine flasks, microporous filter membranes, beakers, pipettes, volumetric flasks, magnetic stirrer, UV spectrophotometer, etc.

2. Materials Fluorouracil, octanol, distilled water, etc.

Experimental Methods

I. Measurement of the Fluorouracil Solubility

1. Determination of the dissolution equilibrium time of drug Weigh about 1g of fluorouracil and put it into the iodine flask, add 50ml of water to it, and put it on a magnetic stirrer to stir and dissolve. After 15, 30, 45, 60, 75, 90, 105, 120, 135, 150min, suck about 3ml of the solution by syringe and filter it through the microporous filter membrane (0.45μm), respectively. Transfer 0.1ml of continuous filtrate in 100ml volumetric flask, and dilute it with water to scale. Measure the absorbance of drug solution at 265nm after mixing the solution evenly. The dissolution equilibrium time is the corresponding time when the solution absorption of two adjacent time points is less than 0.004.

2. Measurement of drug concentration in a saturated solution Take three samples of the solution at an aforementioned equilibrium time point, and filter them through the microporous filter membrane. Take 0.1ml of continuous filtrate in a 100ml volumetric flask, dilute it with water to scale, measure its absorbance at 265nm after mix evenly, and calculate its concentration according to absorbance coefficient ($E_{1cm}^{1\%}$) 522, i.e., fluorouracil solubility.

II. Measurement of the Octanol/Water Partition Coefficient of the Fluorouracil

1. Calculation of the fluorouracil concentration Weigh about 0.5g of fluorouracil, transfer it to an iodine flask, add 100ml of water, shake up, stand for 1h, and suck about 20ml of solution to filter through a microporous filter membrane. Discard the primary filtrate, place the continuous filtrate in a small beaker, and the resulting solution is treated as stock solution. Afterward, suck 0.1ml stock solution into a 100ml volumetric flask, dilute with water to scale, measure the absorbance of the evenly mixed solution at 265nm, and calculate fluorouracil concentration (C) according to absorbance coefficient ($E_{1cm}^{1\%}$) 522.

2. Calculation of the fluorouracil concentration in the water phase Take 10ml of the aforementioned stock solution and transfer it to an iodine flask, add 10ml of octanol, place it on a magnetic stirrer and keep stirring for 1h, stand until layered. Precisely suck 0.1ml of solution at the bottom of iodine flask by pipette, place it in a 100ml volumetric flask, dilute with water to scale, measure the absorbance of the evenly mixed solution at 265nm, and calculate fluorouracil concentration in the water (C_w) according to absorbance coefficient ($E_{1cm}^{1\%}$) 522.

Results and Discussions

1. Solubility of fluorouracil in water

(1) The absorbance of fluorouracil solutions at different time points is recorded in the Table 21–1.

Table 21–1 The absorbance of fluorouracil solutions at different times

Time/min	15	30	45	60	75	90	105	120	135	150
Absorbance (A)										

According to the absorbance value in the table, determine the equilibrium time as_____.

(2) The solubility of fluorouracil solutions at different time points is measured and summarized in the Table 21–2.

Table 21—2　The solubility of fluorouracil in the water

	1	2	3	Mean
Absorbance (A)				
Concentration/(g/100ml)				

2. Measurement of the octanol/water partition coefficient of fluorouracil

(1) The absorbances of the fluorouracil solutions are measured and summarized in the Table 21–3. The average concentration is calculated.

Table 21—3　The mean absorbance and concentration of fluorouracil in the water

	1	2	3	Mean
Absorbance (A)				
Concentration (C)				

(2) The absorbances of fluorouracil in the water after the octanol/water partitioning equilibrium are measured and summarized in the Table 21–4. The average concentration is calculated.

Table 21—4　The mean absorbance and concentration of fluorouracil after the octanol/water partition equilibrium

	1	2	3	Mean
Absorbance (A)				
Concentration (C_w)				

(3) Calculation of the partition coefficient　The octanol/water partition coefficient of fluorouracil is calculated based on the mean of C and C_w.

3. Discussions

(1) Which drug solubility is determined in this experiment? Why?

(2) What are the effects of temperature control on the results of this experiment?

(3) Are there any differences between your results and those obtained by other groups? Please clarify the reason.

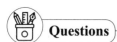 **Questions**

1. What are the main factors affecting drug solubility?

2. What are the differences between the intrinsic solubility and the apparent solubility of the drug?

3. What is the role of the oil/water partition coefficient of drug in the preparation design?

实验二十二　药物的助溶与增溶

 实验目的

1. **掌握**　药物助溶和增溶的原理及影响助溶与增溶的因素。
2. **熟悉**　三相图的绘制及注意事项。

实验原理

　　助溶是指难溶性药物与加入的第三种物质在溶剂中形成可溶性络合物、复盐或缔合物等，以增加药物在溶剂中溶解度的过程，加入的第三种物质称为助溶剂。助溶剂一般为小分子化合物，能溶于水。常用的助溶剂分为两类：一类为有机酸及其钠盐，如苯甲酸钠、水杨酸、对氨基苯甲酸钠等；另一类为酰胺类，如烟酰胺、乌拉坦、尿素等。助溶剂的助溶机制复杂，选择尚无规律可循，一般只能根据药物性质，选择能形成水溶性的络合物、复盐或缔合物的物质作助溶剂。

　　增溶是指某些表面活性剂增大难溶性药物溶解度的作用。具有增溶作用的表面活性剂称为增溶剂，被增溶的物质称为增溶质。增溶的机制为表面活性剂在水中形成胶束，难溶性药物根据自身化学性质，以不同方式与胶束相互作用，分散在胶束中，从而增大其溶解度。常用的增溶剂有聚山梨酯类和聚氧乙烯脂肪酸酯类。增溶剂的种类、用量、药物的性质、加入顺序、温度、pH等均会影响增溶的效果。

　　溶剂－增溶剂－增溶质组成的三组分体系，在恒定的温度和压力下以适宜的比例配制可以得到澄明的溶液，并在稀释时保持澄明。若比例不当，不能得到澄明溶液，或者在稀释时由澄明转为浑浊。通过实验制作三相图是选择溶剂、增溶剂、增溶质正确配比的一种有效方法，可以直观了解物系的状态变化。

实验器材

1. **仪器**　电子天平、滴定管、刻度吸管、烧杯、碘量瓶等。
2. **材料**　茶碱、烟酰胺、乙二胺、薄荷油、聚山梨酯20、蒸馏水等。

实验方法

（一）助溶剂的助溶作用

1. 精密称取茶碱0.198g，放入烧杯中，加水20ml，搅拌5分钟，观察溶解情况。

2. 精密称取茶碱0.198g，烟酰胺0.12g，放入烧杯中，加水20ml，搅拌5分钟，观察溶解情况。

3. 精密称取茶碱0.198g，放入烧杯中，加水19.9ml，滴加乙二胺0.1ml，搅拌5分钟，观察溶解情况。

（二）增溶剂的增溶作用

1. **薄荷油 - 聚山梨酯 20- 蒸馏水三相图绘制** 按表 22-1~ 表 22-3 中所给出的薄荷油 - 聚山梨酯 20- 蒸馏水的质量百分数，在坐标纸上绘出三相图。

表 22-1 区 Ⅰ / Ⅱ 各组分的质量百分数

编号	1	2	3	4	5	6	7	8	9
薄荷油 /%	24.5	30.4	43.8	50.3	55.9	60.0	64.7	71.8	82.5
聚山梨酯 20/%	67.4	64.8	53.6	46.1	41.0	36.7	31.6	26.3	15.1
蒸馏水 /%	8.1	4.8	2.6	3.6	3.1	3.3	3.7	2.9	2.4

表 22-2 区 Ⅱ / Ⅲ 各组分的质量百分数

编号	1	2	3	4	5	6
薄荷油 /%	23.7	25.4	30.8	39.9	46.3	52.6
聚山梨酯 20/%	65.2	62.0	56.5	48.7	42.4	38.6
蒸馏水 /%	11.1	12.6	12.7	11.4	11.3	8.8

表 22-3 区 Ⅲ / Ⅳ 各组分的质量百分数

编号	1	2	3	4	5	6	7	8	9
薄荷油 /%	1.5	3.2	9.0	13.6	19.5	28.2	38.0	43.8	50.4
聚山梨酯 20/%	8.7	16.3	30.3	37.4	41.7	43.2	42.1	40.3	37.0
蒸馏水 /%	89.8	80.5	60.7	49.0	38.8	28.6	19.9	15.9	12.6

2. **不同配比薄荷油 - 聚山梨酯 20 加水量测定** 按表 22-4 中所给出的处方量称量薄荷油与聚山梨酯 20 于碘量瓶中，用滴定管滴加蒸馏水，滴加时轻轻振摇，至出现浑浊时记为终点，观察现象，记录消耗蒸馏水的量。

表 22-4 组分不同配比加水量结果

编号	1	2	3	4
薄荷油 /g	7	3	2	1
聚山梨酯 20/g	3	7	8	9
蒸馏水 /g				

实验结果与讨论

1. **实验结果** 记录上述各实验现象及结果，将不同助溶剂对茶碱的助溶结果及聚山梨酯 20 对薄荷油的增溶结果记录于表 22-5、表 22-6。

表 22-5 不同助溶剂对茶碱的助溶结果

药物	助溶剂	现象
茶碱	无	
茶碱	烟酰胺	
茶碱	乙二胺	

表 22-6　聚山梨酯 20 对薄荷油的增溶结果

编号	1	2	3	4
蒸馏水 /g				
现象				

2. 讨论

（1）讨论烟酰胺和乙二胺对茶碱助溶结果产生差异的可能机制。

（2）在三相图上标出增溶实验中的四种情况所属位置，分析产生不同现象的原因。

思考题

1. 什么是胶束？形成胶束有何意义？

2. 在增溶过程中，增溶剂、药物、溶剂三者以什么顺序混合，增溶效果更好？

3. 影响药物溶解度和溶解速度的因素有哪些？

（张定堃）

Lab. 22　Hydrotropy and Solubilization of Drugs

Experimental Objectives

1. To master the principle and influence factors of hydrotropy and solubilization of drugs.
2. To be familiar with the drawing of three-phase diagram and precautions.

Experimental Principles

Hydrotropy refers to the process in which insoluble drugs form soluble complex, complex salt or association compound between insoluble drugs and the added third substance in the solvent to increase the solubility of drugs in the solvent. The added third substance is called hydrotropic agents. Hydrotropic agents are generally small molecule compounds that are soluble in water. Commonly used hydrotropic agents can be divided into two categories: One is organic acids and their sodium salt, such as sodium benzoate, salicylic acid, sodium p-aminobenzoate, etc.; the other is amide, such as nicotinamide, urethane, urea, etc. The action mechanism of hydrotropy is complex, and the choice of hydrotropic agents is irregular. Generally, we can only choose the substance which can form water-soluble complex, complex salt or association compound as hydrotropic agents according to the property of drugs.

Solubilization refers to the effect of some surfactants to increase the solubility of insoluble drugs. Surfactants with solubilization are called solubilizers, and substances that are solubilized are called solutes. The action mechanism is that surfactants form micelles in water, the insoluble drugs interact with micelles in different ways according to their own chemical properties and disperse in micelles to increase their solubility. Commonly used solubilizers are polysorbate and polyoxyethylene fatty acid esters. The type, dosage of solubilizers, the property of drugs, the order of addition, temperature, and pH will all affect the effect of solubilization.

A three-component system consisting of solvent, solubilizer, and solute can form a clear solution in a proper proportion at a constant temperature and pressure. It has the potential to remain clear when diluted. If the proportion is improper, the clear solution cannot be obtained, or it will turns from clear to cloudy when diluted. It is an effective way that making a three-phase diagram through experiments to select the proper proportion of solvent, solubilizer, and solute, which can directly understand the state change of the system.

Equipments and Materials

1. **Equipments**　Electronic balance, burette, graduated pipette, beaker, iodine measuring bottle, etc.
2. **Materials**　Theophylline, nicotinamide, ethylenediamine, peppermint oil, polysorbate 20,

distilled water, etc.

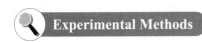 **Experimental Methods**

I. Hydrotropy Effect of Hydrotropic Agents

1. 0.198g of theophylline was precisely weighed and put into a beaker. Add 20ml of water, stir for 5min, and observe the dissolution.

2. 0.198g of theophylline and 0.12g of nicotinamide were precisely weighed and put into a beaker. Add 20ml of water, stir for 5min, and observe the dissolution.

3. 0.198g of theophylline was precisely weighed and put into a beaker. Add 20ml of water and 0.1ml of ethylenediamine, stir for 5min, and observe the dissolution.

II. Solubilization Effect of Solubilizers

1. Drawing of three-phase diagram of peppermint oil- polysorbate 20-distilled water. According to the mass percentages of peppermint oil- polysorbate 20-water given in the Table 22–1 to Table 22–3, draw the three-phase diagram on the coordinate paper.

Table 22–1 Mass percent of components I / II

Number	1	2	3	4	5	6	7	8	9
Peppermint oil/%	24.5	30.4	43.8	50.3	55.9	60.0	64.7	71.8	82.5
Polysorbate 20/%	67.4	64.8	53.6	46.1	41.0	36.7	31.6	26.3	15.1
Distilled water/%	8.1	4.8	2.6	3.6	3.1	3.3	3.7	2.9	2.4

Table 22–2 Mass percent of components II / III

Number	1	2	3	4	5	6
Peppermint oil/%	23.7	25.4	30.8	39.9	46.3	52.6
Polysorbate 20/%	65.2	62.0	56.5	48.7	42.4	38.6
Distilled water/%	11.1	12.6	12.7	11.4	11.3	8.8

Table 22–3 Mass percent of components III / IV

Number	1	2	3	4	5	6	7	8	9
Peppermint oil/%	1.5	3.2	9.0	13.6	19.5	28.2	38.0	43.8	50.4
Polysorbate 20/%	8.7	16.3	30.3	37.4	41.7	43.2	42.1	40.3	37.0
Distilled water/%	89.8	80.5	60.7	49.0	38.8	28.6	19.9	15.9	12.6

2. Determination of water addition amount of peppermint oil-polysorbate 20 in different proportions. Weigh the peppermint oil and polysorbate 20 into the iodine measuring bottle according to the prescription given in the Table 22–4. Add distilled water with burette, shake gently when dropping, and record the end point when turbidity appears. Observe the phenomenon and record the consumption of distilled water.

Table 22-4   Water addition results for different components

Number	1	2	3	4
Peppermint oil/g	7	3	2	1
polysorbate 20/g	3	7	8	9
Distilled water/g				

 Results and Discussions

1. Results   Record the above experimental phenomena and results. The hydrotropy results of theophylline with different hydrotropic agents are listed in the Table 22-5. The solubilization results of peppermint oil with polysorbate 20 are listed in the Table 22-6.

Table 22-5   Hydrotropy results of theophylline by different hydrotropic agents

Drug	Hydrotropic agent	Phenomena
Theophylline	\	
Theophylline	Nicotinamide	
Theophylline	Ethylenediamine	

Table 22-6   Solubilization results of polysorbate 20 on peppermint oil

Number	1	2	3	4
Distilled water/g				
Phenomena				

2. Discussions

(1) Try to discuss the possible mechanisms of the hydrotropy result difference between nicotinamide and ethylenediamine with theophylline.

(2) Mark the positions of four conditions in solubilization experiment on the three-phase diagram, and analyze the causes of different phenomena.

Questions

1. What is the micelles? What is the significance of forming micelles?

2. During the process of solubilization, in what order are the solubilizers, drugs, and solvents mixed to achieve a better solubilization effect?

3. What are the factors that affect the solubility and dissolution rate of drugs?

实验二十三　粉体的粒径与粒度分布的测定

实验目的

1. **掌握**　筛分法测定粉体粒度分布的原理和方法。
2. **了解**　根据筛分数据绘制粒度频率分布曲线和累积分布曲线的方法和意义。

实验原理

　　粒径是粒子的大小，粒度分布通常是指某一粒径或粒径范围的颗粒在整个粉体中所占的比例，可用简单的表格、绘图和函数形式表示颗粒群粒径的分布状态。粒径、粒度分布能显著影响粉体及其产品的性质及加工性能，如颗粒的凝结时间、颗粒的强度、粉体的流动性、混合、制粒、压片等。为了控制药物制剂生产过程以保证产品合格，在生产过程中必须及时取样并对产品进行粒度分布的检验，粉碎和分级也需要测量粒度。粒度测定方法有多种，常用的有筛分法、沉降法、激光法、库尔特计数仪法、吸附法等，对于不规则的粒子，其粒径的测定方法不同，物理意义也不同。本实验采用筛分法测定粉体粒度分布。

　　筛分法是应用最广泛的粒度测定方法之一，利用筛分方法不仅可以测定粒度分布，而且通过绘制累积粒度特性曲线，还可得到累积产率 50% 时的平均粒度。筛分法是让粉体样品通过一系列不同筛孔的标准筛，将其分离成若干个粒级，分别称重，求得以质量百分数表示的粒度分布。筛分法适用于测量 20μm~100mm 之间的粒度分布；如果采用电成型筛（微孔筛），其筛孔尺寸可小至 5μm，甚至更小。筛孔的大小习惯上用"目"表示，其含义是每英寸（2.54cm）长度上筛孔的数目，也有用 1cm 长度上的孔数或 1cm² 筛面上的孔数表示的，也有直接以筛孔的尺寸来表示。筛分法常使用符合《中国药典》规定的标准套筛。

　　筛分法有干法与湿法两种，测定粒度分布时，一般用干法筛分，若试样含水较多、颗粒凝聚性较强时则应当用湿法筛分。特别是颗粒较细的物料，若允许与水混合时，最好使用湿法。因为湿法可避免微细粉粒附着在筛孔上而堵塞筛孔。另外，湿法不受物料温度和大气湿度的影响，还可以改善操作条件。湿法与干法均已被列为国家标准方法。

　　筛分法除了常用的手筛分、机械筛分、湿法筛分外，还采用空气筛分、声筛分、淘筛分和自组筛分等，其筛分结果往往采用频率分布和累积分布来表示颗粒的粒度分布。频率分布表示各个粒径相对应的颗粒百分含量（微分型）；累积分布表示小于（或大于）某粒径的颗粒占全部颗粒的百分含量与该粒径的关系（积分型）。常用表格或图形来直观表示颗粒粒径的频率分布和累积分布。

实验器材

1. **仪器**　天平、标准药筛、振筛机、烘箱、搪瓷盘等。
2. **材料**　碳酸氢钠、滑石粉等。

实验方法

（一）粉末筛分

1. 准确称取已烘干的碳酸氢钠、滑石粉各 200g 样品。

2. 将标准筛按孔径由大至小的顺序叠好，并装上筛底，将称好的试样倒入最上层筛子，加上筛盖，安装在振筛机上。

3. 开动振筛机，振动 10 分钟，取下筛子。用手筛分，若 1 分钟所得筛下物料量小于物料的 1%，则已达筛分终点，否则要继续手筛至终点。

4. 分别称量各筛上和底盘中的试样质量，记录数据于表 23-1 中。

5. 检查各层筛面质量总和与原试样质量之差，误差不应超过 2%，此时可把所损失的质量加在最细粒级中；若误差超过 2% 时，需重新进行实验。

【注意事项】如没有振筛机，可用手均匀摇振筛子，每分钟拍打 120 次，每拍打 25 次将筛子转 1/8 圈，使试样分散在筛布上，拍打约 10 分钟，直至筛分终点（终点时拍打 1 分钟后筛下物小于筛上物料的 1%）。

（二）记录数据

将标准筛中各级粉末称定质量，记录于表 23-1。

表 23-1　粉体筛分分级结果

标准筛		筛上粉末重量 /g	分级质量百分率 /%	筛上累积百分率 /%	筛下累积百分率 /%
筛号	筛孔大小 /μm				
1	2000±70				
2	850±29				
3	355±13				
4	250±9.9				
5	180±7.6				
6	150±6.6				
7	125±5.8				
8	90±4.6				
9	75±4.1				
底盘	0				
合计					

实验结果与讨论

1. 数据处理

（1）计算实验误差　检查各层筛面质量总和与原试样质量之误差：

$$实验误差 = \frac{试样质量 - 筛分总质量}{试样质量} \times 100\% \qquad (23\text{-}1)$$

误差不应超过 2%，此时可把所损失的质量加在最细粒级中。若误差超过 2% 时，应另取试样，重新进行实验。

（2）绘制曲线　根据实验结果，在直角毫米坐标纸上绘图表示颗粒群粒径的分布状态，也可用 Excel 作图。根据实验结果记录，在坐标纸上绘制筛上累积分布曲线 R，筛下累积分布曲线 D。

（3）分析　一个药筛的各个筛孔可以看作是一个系列的量轨，当颗粒处于筛孔上，有的颗粒可以通过而有的通不过。颗粒位于一筛孔处的概率由下列因素决定：颗粒大小分布、筛面上颗粒的数量、颗粒的物理性质（如表面积）、药筛振动的方法、药筛表面的几何形状（如开口面积 / 总面积）等。位于筛孔上的颗粒是否能通过则取决于颗粒的尺寸和颗粒在筛面上的角度。

筛分所测得的颗粒大小分布还取决于下列因素：筛分的持续时间、筛孔的偏差、筛子的磨损、观察和实验误差、取样误差、不同筛子和不同操作的影响等。

2. 讨论

（1）对物料进行筛分时，物料哪些性质对筛分效率有较大的影响？在实验前应对试样如何处理，使之达到实验要求？

（2）实验过程中可能产生误差的环节有哪些？如何避免或减小误差？

思考题

1. 试分析颗粒大小与颗粒吸湿性、流动性的关系。

2. 干筛法测定颗粒粒度分布的影响因素有哪些？

3. 粒度测定方法有哪些？各自的特点及适用范围是什么？

（王文苹）

Lab. 23 Particle Size and Size Distribution Test of Powders

 Experimental Objectives

1. To learn the principles and methods for determination on particle size distribution of powder by the sieving method.

2. To understand the method and significance of frequency or cumulative distribution curves based on sieving data.

 Experimental Principles

Particle size means the dimensions of particles. Size distribution generally refers to the percentage ratio of particles within a specific size range in the whole powder material, and can be expressed as simple table, plot or function. Both particle size and size distribution can significantly influence the property and processability of the powder and its products, such as aggregation time of particles, particle strength, flowability of powder, mixing, granulating and tableting process, etc. To control the manufacturing process and ensure the quality of pharmaceutical products, particle size distribution test is required during the grinding, grading and production processes. There are many approaches to determine size distribution of powders, and commonly used methods include sieving, sedimentation, laser, Coulter counting, adsorption, etc. For particles with irregular shape, different test methods stand for different physical meaning. The sieving method is adopted in the present experiment to measure the particle size distribution.

Sieving is the most commonly used method for determination of particle size. And the average particle size at 50% of cumulative yield can also be calculated by plotting cumulative curves of particle size after sieving. This method passes a powder specimen through a series of standard sieves with different opening size to obtain several particle fractions with related size, weighs the particle fractions and then calculate the size distribution expressed as weight percentage composition. The sieving method is suitable for size distribution determination of particles within a range of 20μm~100mm. The opening size of electroforming sieve (i.e. micromesh) can be as tiny as 5μm, or even smaller. The size of sieve opening is customarily expressed as "mesh", which means the opening number on 2.54cm length of the sieve. Sometimes the "mesh" represents the opening number on 1cm length or 1cm^2 area of the sieve, or directly shows as the size of the sieve opening. The standard sieves in accordance with the requirements of *Chinese Pharmacopoeia* are commonly used for the sieving method.

There are two types of sieving methods, dry sieving and wet sieving. Dry sieving method is generally applied for determination of size distribution. Wet sieving method is for the specimen with much water content and strong flocculation of particles, especially for fine powders with permission to mix with

172

water. Wet sieving method can avoid the adhesion of fine powders onto the opening and blockage of the sieve mesh, and can prevent the influence of material temperature and atmosphere humidity. Both dry and wet sieving are listed as national standard methods.

Except for commonly used hand-sieving, mechanical sieving and wet sieving methods, other methods (such as air jet sieving, sonic sieving, panning, self-screening) are also included. The sieving results are usually presented as frequency distribution or cumulative distribution to express the particle size distribution. The frequency distribution means percentage composition of particles in a specific size range (in a differential form). The cumulative distribution means the relation between the particle size larger or smaller than a specific value and the percentage composition of the corresponding particles (in an intcgral form). Tables or graphs are usually applied to describe the frequency or cumulative distribution of particle size.

 Equipments and Materials

1. **Equipments**   Balance, standard sieves, sieve shaker, air oven, enameled tray, etc.
2. **Materials**   Sodium bicarbonate, talc, etc.

 Experimental Methods

I. Sieving of Fine Powders

【Procedure】

(1) Accurately weigh out 200g of sodium bicarbonate and talc, respectively.

(2) Assemble a nest of sieves on the receiving pan in an order of decreasing opening size. Place the specimen on the uppermost sieve, cover with a lid, and then install on the sieve shaker.

(3) Run the shaker for 10min, and then shake the sieves by hand. Endpoint will be reached when the powder amount under the sieves is less than 1% of the total specimen. Keeping sieving by hand until reaching the endpoint.

(4) Weigh the amount remaining on each sieve and in the receiving pan, then fill the results into the Table 23-1.

(5) The weight change of the specimen before and after sieving must not exceed 2% of the weight of the original specimen. The total loss can be added on the finest powders. The whole procedure must be repeated when the weight change is over 2%.

【Note】Hand-shaking process can be applied when there is no sieving shaker. Flap the sieves for 10min at 120 times per minute and turn the sieves for 1/8 circle every 25 times. Keep taping until reaching the endpoint.

II. Record the Data

Fill the weight of the remaining powders into the Table 23-1.

Table 23-1   Grading result of powders by sieving

Standard sieve		Powder weight on the sieve/g	Grading weight percentage/%	Accumulative percentage on the sieve/%	Accumulative percentage under the sieve/%
Sieve No.	Opening diameter/μm				
1	2000±70				
2	850±29				

Continued

Standard sieve		Powder weight on the sieve/g	Grading weight percentage/%	Accumulative percentage on the sieve/%	Accumulative percentage under the sieve/%
Sieve No.	Opening diameter/μm				
3	355±13				
4	250±9.9				
5	180±7.6				
6	150±6.6				
7	125±5.8				
8	90±4.6				
9	75±4.1				
Receiving pan	0				
Sum					

 Results and Discussions

1. Data analysis

(1) Calculate the test deviation. Check any difference between the initial specimen weight and the total specimen weight on the sieves.

$$\text{Experimental Error} = \frac{\text{Original specimen weight} - \text{Total weight after sieving}}{\text{Original specimen weight}} \times 100\%$$

The weight change of the specimen before and after sieving must not exceed 2% of the weight of the original specimen. The total loss can be added on the finest powders. The whole procedure must be repeated when the weight change is over 2%.

(2) Plot the curves. According to the experimental results, plot the particle size distribution data on a piece of rectangular millimeter coordinate paper or by the EXCEL on a computer. And draw the accumulative distribution curve on the sieve (*R*) and under the sieve (*D*), respectively.

(3) Analyze the data. Each opening of a sieve mesh can be regarded as a series of measuring rail. When we place the specimen on the sieve mesh, some particles can pass through the opening while the others cannot. The probability for one particle to locate in an opening of the sieve is depended on the following factors: particle size distribution, the particle numbers on the sieve mesh, the physical properties of the particles (e.g. surface area), shaking method for the sieve, geometric shape of sieve surface (i.e. the ratio between opening area and total area), etc. Whether the particle on the sieve can pass through the opening or not rely on the size and shape of the particle, and the angle between the particle and the sieve as well.

The test result of particle size distribution by the sieving method is also depended on the factors below: duration time of sieving, deviation on opening size of sieves, abrasion condition of sieves, error of observation, test error, error of sampling, different sieves and operation, etc.

2. Discussions

(1) Describe the material properties which act more effect on the sieving efficiency. And find out the pretreatment method for the test specimen to meet the experimental requirements.

(2) Which procedure may result in any experimental error during the whole process? And how to

avoid or minimize the errors?

 Questions

1. What is the relation between particle size and its moisture absorption or flowability?
2. What are the influencing factors for particle size distribution test by the dry sieving method?
3. Describe the test methods for particle size determination and their features and application.

实验二十四　粉体流动性的测定

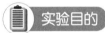

实验目的

1. **掌握**　常用粉体流动性参数的测定方法。
2. **熟悉**　影响粉体流动性的因素及改善方法。
3. **了解**　粉体润滑剂、助流剂的助流原理。

实验原理

　　粉体的流动性直接影响制剂的质量，是固体制剂制备过程中必须考察的重要性质之一。粉体粒子间的作用力（如范德华力、静电力等）、粒度与粒度分布、粒子形态及表面摩擦力等多种因素均会影响粉体的流动性。休止角、流出速度和压缩度是表征粉体流动性的常用指标，其中前两者表示粉体在重力作用下的流动性，后者则表示粉体在振荡力作用下的流动性。加入润滑剂或助流剂（如滑石粉、微粉硅胶等）是改善粉体流动性的常用方法，其通过混合过程附着于粉体表面，减弱粒子间的黏着从而增强粉体流动性，增大充填密度。

　　休止角是指粉体堆积形成的自由斜面上粒子所受重力和粒子间摩擦力达到平衡并处于静止状态时与水平面所形成的夹角（θ）。常用的测定方法有固定圆锥法、固定漏斗法、倾斜箱法、转动圆筒法等，其中固定圆锥法最为常用。一般认为，$\theta \leqslant 30°$ 时流动性较好，$\theta \leqslant 40°$ 时可以满足生产过程中的流动性需求。值得注意的是，休止角随测量方法的不同所得数据差异较大，重现性较差，因此不能将其作为粉体的物理常数。

　　流出速度是指粉体由一定孔径的孔或管中流出的速度，流出速度越快，粉体流动性越好，它主要反应粉体的粒度和均匀度。如果粉体的流动性差而不能流出时，可加入直径 100μm 的玻璃球助流，测定粉体自由流动所需玻璃球的最少加入量（$w\%$），最少加入量越大则流动性越差。

　　压缩度是指粉体在振动前后的堆积密度的变化百分率。其反应振动状态下粉体的流动性。压缩度在 20% 以下时流动性较好，当压缩度达到 40%~50% 时粉体很难从容器中流出。

　　本实验通过测定不同粉体的上述流动性参数，考察粒子大小、形状和助流剂对粉体流动性的影响。

实验器材

1. **仪器**　休止角测定仪、流出速度测定仪、粉体振动仪（或粉体综合特性测定仪）等。
2. **材料**　微晶纤维素微球、微晶纤维素粉末（中粉、极细粉）、滑石粉、硬脂酸镁、微粉硅胶、玻璃球（$\Phi=100\mu m$）等。

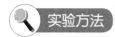 实验方法

（一）休止角的测定

如图 24-1 所示，将待测物料均匀地注入圆盘中心，直至物料形成圆锥体并沿圆盘边缘自由落下为止，测定圆盘半径（R）和圆锥体高度（H），按照公式（24-1）计算休止角；或用量角器测定休止角。

$$\tan\theta=H/R \qquad\qquad (24\text{-}1)$$

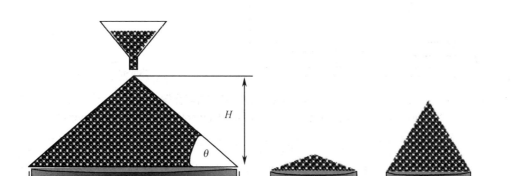

图 24-1 休止角测定装置示意图

Figure 24-1 Schematic diagram of angle of repose measuring device

【实验过程】

（1）分别准确称取微晶纤维素微球、微晶纤维素中粉和微晶纤维素极细粉各 50.0g，测定休止角，平行测定三次，比较物料的形状、粒径大小对休止角的影响。

（2）分别准确称取微晶纤维素中粉各 50.0g，共 3 份，分别向其中加入 1.0% 的滑石粉、微粉硅胶和硬脂酸镁，混合均匀后测定休止角，平行测定三次，比较三种润滑剂的助流效果。

（3）分别准确称取微晶纤维素中粉各 50.0g，共 6 份，分别向其中加入 0、0.5%、1.0%、2.0%、5.0% 和 10.0% 的滑石粉，均匀混合后测定其休止角，比较滑石粉用量对流动性的影响。以休止角为纵坐标，滑石粉用量为横坐标，绘制曲线，选择滑石粉最适宜的加入量。

【注意事项】

（1）为了使待测物料落至圆盘中心，应使漏斗下端出口正对圆盘中心，将物料从漏斗上部缓缓加入。

（2）如果物料流动性差而不易从漏斗流出时，可在漏斗上部放一网筛（16~18 目），边过筛边加入，必要时适当轻敲网筛和漏斗。

（二）流出速度的测定

如图 24-2 所示，将一定量的待测物料装入流出速度测定仪（或三角漏斗中），打开下部流出口滑门，测定全部物料流出所需时间。

【实验过程】

（1）分别准确称取微晶纤维素微球、微晶纤维素中粉和微晶纤维素极细粉各 20.0g，测定流出速度，平行测定三次，比较物料的形状和粒径大小对流出速度的影响。

（2）准确称取微晶纤维素中粉 20.0g，共 3 份，分别向其中加入 1.0% 的滑石粉、微粉硅胶和硬脂酸镁，混合均匀后测定流出速度，平行测定三次，比较三种润滑剂的助流效果。

（3）分别准确称取微晶纤维素中粉各 20.0g，共 6 份，分别向其中加入 0、0.5%、1.0%、

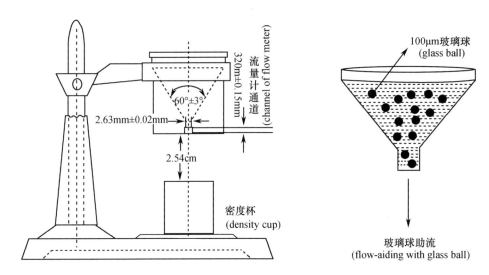

图 24-2 流出速度测定装置示意图

Figure 24-2　Schematic diagram of the efflux velocity measuring device

2.0%、5.0% 和 10.0% 的滑石粉，混合均匀后测定流出速度，比较滑石粉用量对流动性的影响。以流出速度为纵坐标，滑石粉用量为横坐标，绘制曲线，选择滑石粉最适宜的加入量。

（4）分别准确称取微晶纤维素中粉与微晶纤维素极细粉各 50.0g，分别向其中加入 10% 的 100μm 玻璃球助流，平行测定三次，比较加入前后对粉体流出速度的影响。

（三）压缩度的测定

取约 30g 待测物料，精密称定，加入量筒中，测量体积，计算松密度 ρ_{b}。将量筒装入粉体振动仪中进行轻敲（频率 250Hz·min^{-1}、幅度 3.0mm ± 0.2mm），直至体积不变（$RSD \leqslant 2\%$）为止，测量最终体积，计算振实密度 ρ_{bt}，按照公式（24-2）计算压缩度 C。

$$C = \frac{\rho_{bt} - \rho_{b}}{\rho_{b}} \times 100\% \tag{24-2}$$

【实验过程】

（1）分别准确称取 30.0g 的微晶纤维素微球、微晶纤维素中粉和微晶纤维素极细粉，测定压缩度，平行测定三次，比较物料的形状和粒径大小对压缩度的影响。

（2）分别准确称取微晶纤维素中粉各 30.0g，共 3 份，分别向其中加入 1.0% 的滑石粉、微粉硅胶和硬脂酸镁，均匀混合后测定压缩度，平行测定三次，比较不同润滑剂对压缩度的影响。

（3）分别准确称取微晶纤维素中粉各 20.0g，共 6 份，分别向其中加入 0、0.5%、1.0%、2.0%、5.0% 和 10.0% 的滑石粉，混合均匀后测定压缩度，比较滑石粉用量对压缩度的影响。以压缩度为纵坐标，滑石粉用量为横坐标，绘出曲线，选择滑石粉最适宜的加入量。

💬 **实验结果与讨论**

1. 结果　请将实验结果依次填入表 24-1 至表 24-3；根据表 24-2 实验结果，绘制"滑石粉用量-流动性参数"曲线图。

表 24-1　不同物料和润滑剂的流动性参数

因素 1		休止角 /°				流出速度 /（g/s）				压缩度 /%			
		1	2	3	$\bar{x}$	1	2	3	$\bar{x}$	1	2	3	$\bar{x}$
物料	微晶纤维素微球												
	微晶纤维素中粉												
	微晶纤维素极细粉												
润滑剂	滑石粉												
	微粉硅胶												
	硬脂酸镁												

表 24-2　滑石粉加入量对流动性参数的影响

流动性参数	滑石粉加入量 /%					
	0	0.5	1.0	2.0	5.0	10.0
休止角 /°						
流出速度 /（g/s）						
压缩度 /%						

表 24-3　玻璃球对物料流动速度的影响

物料	加入玻璃球之前流出速度 /（g/s）				加入玻璃球之后流出速度 /（g/s）			
	1	2	3	$\bar{x}$	1	2	3	$\bar{x}$
微晶纤维素中粉								
微晶纤维素极细粉								

2. 讨论

（1）比较微晶纤维素微球、微晶纤维素中粉、微晶纤维素极细粉的流动性大小并分析原因。

（2）不同润滑剂对微晶纤维素中粉的流动性有何影响？是否润滑剂用量越大，流动性越好？

（3）比较玻璃球与润滑剂对微晶纤维素中粉流动性的影响。

📝 思考题

1. 影响粉体流动性的因素有哪些？列举能够改善粉体流动性的措施。

2. 润滑剂和助流剂的作用机制有何不同？

3. 评价粉体流动性的指标有哪些？各有何特点？

（邹俊波）

Lab.24　Determination of Powder Fluidity

 Experimental Objectives

1. To master the determination methods of common powder fluidity parameters.
2. To be familiar with the factors affecting the fluidity of powder and the improvement methods.
3. To understand the flow-aiding principle of lubricant and glidants.

 Experimental Principles

The fluidity of the powder directly affects the quality of the preparation which is one of the important properties that must be investigated in the preparation of solid preparation. The fluidity of powder is affected by many factors, such as interaction force between powder particles (such as van der Waals force, electrostatic force, etc.), particle size and particle size distribution, particle morphology, surface friction and so on. Angle of repose, efflux velocity and compressibility are commonly used indexes to characterize the fluidity of powder, in which the first two represent the fluidity of powder under the action of gravity, and the latter indicate the fluidity of powder under the action of oscillating force. The addition of lubricants or glidants (such as talc powder, siliciidoxydum, etc.) is a common method to improve the fluidity of powders, which adheres to the surface of powders through the mixing process, weakens the adhesion between particles, so as to enhance the fluidity of powders and increase the filling density.

The angle of repose refers to the angle (θ) between the oblique plane and the horizontal plane at rest when the gravity and friction between the particles on the free slope formed by the accumulation of powder are balanced. The commonly used determination methods include fixed cone method, fixed funnel method, inclined box method, rotating cylinder method and so on, among which the fixed cone method is the most commonly used. It is generally believed that the fluidity is ideal when $\theta \leqslant 30°$, while $\theta \leqslant 40°$ satisfies the liquidity requirements in the production process. It is worth noting that the angle of repose varies greatly with different measurement methods which leads to its poor reproducibility, so it cannot be regarded as the physical constant of the powder.

The efflux velocity refers to the speed at which the powder flows out of a hole or tube with a certain aperture. The faster the efflux speed is, the better the fluidity of the powder is. It mainly reflects the particle size and uniformity of the powder. Glass balls with a diameter of 100μm can be added to assist fluidity of the powder when it is too poor to flow out. The minimum amount of glass ball ($w\%$) required for the free flow of the powder can be used to determine the fluidity. The greater the minimum amount, the worse the fluidity.

The compressibility refers to the percentage change of the bulk density of the powder before and after vibration which reflects the fluidity of the powder under the oscillating force. It is ideal when the compressibility is less than 20% while 40% ~ 50% makes it difficult for the powder to flow out of the container.

In this laboratory, the effects of particle size, shape and glidants on the fluidity of different powders will be investigated by measuring the above fluidity parameters of different powders.

 Equipments and Materials

1. Equipments Angle of repose tester, efflux velocity tester, powder vibrator (or powder comprehensive characteristic tester), etc.

2. Materials Microcrystalline cellulose microsphere, microcrystalline cellulose powder (medium powder, ultra-fine powder), talc powder, magnesium stearate, siliciidoxydum, glass ball (Φ=100μm), etc.

 Experimental Methods

I. Determination of the Angle of Repose

As shown in the Figure 24–1, the powder to be tested is uniformly injected into the center of the disc until the material forms a cone and falls freely along the edge of the disc, the radius of the disc (R) and the height of the cone (H), are calculated according to the Formula 24–1, or the angle of repose is measured by a protractor.

$$\tan \theta = H/R \tag{24-1}$$

【Procedure】

(1) Weigh accurately a quantity equivalent to about 50.0g of microcrystalline cellulose microspheres, microcrystalline cellulose medium powder and microcrystalline cellulose ultra-fine powder respectively, measure the angle of repose for three times in parallel, compare the effects of material shape and particle size on the angle of repose.

(2) Weigh accurately a quantity equivalent to about 50.0g of microcrystalline cellulose medium powder in triplicate, and 1.0% talcum powder, micro powder silica gel and magnesium stearate are added respectively, measure the angle of repose three times in parallel after mixing evenly, compare the flow-aiding effects of the three kinds of lubricants.

(3) Weigh accurately a quantity of microcrystalline cellulose medium powder equivalent to about 50.0g each for a total of 6 parts into which adding 0, 0.5%, 1.0%, 2.0%, 5.0% and 10.0% talc powder respectively, compare the effect of talc powder dosage on fluidity by determining the angle of repose after mixing evenly, draw the curve with the angle of repose as the ordinate and the amount of talc as the abscissa from which we can select the most suitable amount of talc powder for flow-aiding.

【Notes】

(1) In order to make the material to be tested fall to the center of the disc, the lower outlet of the funnel should be directly facing the center of the disc, and the material should be added slowly from the upper part of the funnel.

(2) It is necessary for sieving the powder (with 16~18 mesh sieve) on the top of the funnel if the fluidity of the material is poor or hard to flow out. Appropriately tapping the sieve and funnel if necessary is also advised.

II. Determination of Efflux Velocity

As shown in the Figure 24–2, the material to be tested is loaded into the efflux velocity tester (or triangular funnel), and the sliding door of the lower outlet is opened to determine the time required for all materials to flow out.

【Procedure】

(1) Weigh accurately a quantity equivalent to about 20.0g of microcrystalline cellulose microspheres, microcrystalline cellulose medium powder and microcrystalline cellulose ultra-fine powder respectively, measure the efflux velocity for three times in parallel, compare the effects of material shape and particle size on the efflux velocity.

(2) Weigh accurately a quantity of microcrystalline cellulose medium powder equivalent to about 20.0g each for a total of 3 parts into which adding 1.0% talc powder, siliciidoxydum and magnesium stearate respectively, compare the flow-aiding effects of the three lubricants by measuring the efflux velocity after mixing evenly.

(3) Weigh accurately a quantity of microcrystalline cellulose medium powder equivalent to about 20.0g each for a total of 6 parts into which adding 0, 0.5%, 1.0%, 2.0%, 5.0% and 10.0% talc powder respectively, compare the effect of talc powder dosage on fluidity by determining the efflux velocity after mixing evenly, draw the curve with the efflux velocity as the ordinate and the amount of talc as the abscissa from which we can select the most suitable amount of talc powder for flow-aiding.

(4) Weigh accurately a quantity equivalent to about 50.0g of microcrystalline cellulose medium powder and microcrystalline cellulose ultra-fine powder respectively into which 10% glass ball ($\Phi = 100\mu m$) are added to aid flow, compare the effects before and after adding on the efflux velocity of the powder after three times of parallel measurement.

III. Determination of Compressibility

Weigh accurately a quantity equivalent to about 30.0g powder in the measuring cylinder, measure the volume and calculate the loose density ρ_b. The measuring cylinder is loaded into the powder vibrometer and tapped (frequency 250Hz·min^{-1}, amplitude 3.0mm±0.2mm), until the volume is constant ($RSD \leqslant 2\%$) from which we can get the tap density ρ_{bt} by measuring the final volume. Compressibility C is calculated according to the Formula 24-2.

$$C = \frac{\rho_{bt} - \rho_b}{\rho_b} \times 100\%$$ (24-2)

【Procedure】

(1) Weigh accurately a quantity equivalent to about 30.0g of microcrystalline cellulose microspheres, microcrystalline cellulose medium powder and microcrystalline cellulose ultra-fine powder respectively, measure the compressibility for three times in parallel, compare the effects of material shape and particle size on the compressibility.

(2) Weigh accurately a quantity of microcrystalline cellulose medium powder equivalent to about 30.0g each for a total of 3 parts into which adding 1.0% talc powder, siliciidoxydum and magnesium stearate respectively, compare the flow-aiding effects of the three lubricants by measuring the compressibility after mixing evenly.

(3) Weigh accurately a quantity of microcrystalline cellulose medium powder equivalent to about 20.0g each for a total of 6 parts into which adding 0, 0.5%, 1.0%, 2.0%, 5.0% and 10.0% talc powder respectively, compare the effect of talc powder dosage on fluidity by determining the compressibility after mixing evenly, draw the curve with the compressibility as the ordinate and the amount of talc as the abscissa from which we can select the most suitable amount of glidants for flow-aiding.

Results and Discussion

1. Results Please fill the experimental results in the Table 24–1 to the Table 24–3 in turn, and draw the curve of "talc dosage-fluidity parameters" according to the experimental results of the Table 24–2.

Table 24–1 Fluidity parameters of different materials and glidants

Factors 1		Angle of repose/°				Efflux velocity/(g/s)				Compressibility/%			
		1	2	3	$\bar{x}$	1	2	3	$\bar{x}$	1	2	3	$\bar{x}$
Materials	Microcrystalline cellulose microspheres												
	Microcrystalline cellulose medium powder												
	Microcrystalline cellulose ultra-fine powder												
Glidants	Talc powder												
	Siliciidoxydum												
	Magnesium stearate												

Table 24–2 The affecting of the amount of talc powder added on fluidity parameters

Fluidity parameters	The amount of talc powder added/%					
	0	0.5	1.0	2.0	5.0	10.0
Angle of repose/°						
Efflux velocity/(g/s)						
Compressibility/%						

Table 24–3 The effects of glass ball adding on the efflux velocity

Materials	Efflux velocity before adding glass balls/(g/s)				Efflux velocity after adding glass balls/(g/s)			
	1	2	3	$\bar{x}$	1	2	3	$\bar{x}$
Microcrystalline cellulose medium powder								
Microcrystalline cellulose ultra-fine powder								

2. Discussions

(1) Compare the fluidity of microcrystalline cellulose microsphere, microcrystalline cellulose medium powder and microcrystalline cellulose ultra-fine powder and analyze the reasons.

(2) What is the effect of different lubricants on the fluidity of microcrystalline cellulose medium powder? Is it true that the greater the amount of lubricant, the better the fluidity?

(3) Compare the effect of glass ball and lubricant on the fluidity of microcrystalline cellulose medium powder.

Questions

1. What are the factors that affect the fluidity of powder? List some measures that can improve the fluidity of powder.

2. What is the difference between lubricants and glidants?

3. What are the indicators to evaluate the fluidity of powders? What are the characteristics of each?

实验二十五　粉体吸湿性的测定

PPT

实验目的

1. **掌握**　水（不）溶性药物及其混合物的吸湿特性。
2. **熟悉**　吸湿平衡曲线的绘制方法及临界相对湿度的测定方法。
3. **了解**　影响粉体吸湿性和吸湿速度的因素及改善措施。

实验原理

吸湿是指固体表面吸附水分的现象。将药物粉末置于湿度较大的空气中时容易发生不同程度的吸湿现象，以使粉末的流动性下降、固结、润湿、液化等，甚至促进化学反应而降低药物的稳定性。

粉体的吸湿性与空气湿度有关，在较大湿度的空气中易吸湿（吸潮），在干空气中易被干燥（风干），直至吸湿与干燥达到动态平衡，此时的含水量称为平衡水分。空气的相对湿度（relative humidity, RH）是空气中水蒸气分压与同温度下饱和空气水蒸气分压之比，是反映空气状态的重要参数。通常空气的相对湿度在 0~100% 之间。若将粉体在不同相对湿度空气环境下的平衡吸湿量对相对湿度作图，即得吸湿平衡曲线，该曲线可反映出粉体的吸湿特性。药物原料以及其他制剂粉体的吸湿特性主要取决于粉体自身的性质。

1. 水溶性物料的吸湿性　水溶性的粉体在较低的相对湿度环境中其平衡水分含量较低，不吸湿，但当空气中的相对湿度提高到某一定值时，吸湿量急剧增加，此时的相对湿度称为粉体的临界相对湿度（critical relative humidity, CRH）。CRH 是水溶性药物固有的特征参数，CRH 越小则表明药物越易吸湿。为了防止物料的吸湿，应确保操作环境和贮存环境空气湿度在 CRH 以下。

根据 Elder 假说，水溶性物料 A 和 B 混合物的 CRH_{AB} 约等于两组分 CRH 的乘积，而与组分的量无关，即 $CRH_{AB}=CRH_A \cdot CRH_B$。表明水溶性物料混合物的 CRH 值低于其中任何一种物料的 CRH 值，因而更易于吸湿。

2. 水不溶性物料的吸湿性　水不溶性物料的吸湿性在相对湿度变化时缓慢发生变化，没有临界点。由于平衡水分吸附在固体表面，相当于水分的等温吸附曲线。水不溶性物料混合物的吸湿性具有加和性，即 $CRH_{AB}=CRH_A + CRH_B$。

实验器材

1. **仪器**　分析天平、干燥器、恒温箱、称量瓶等。
2. **材料**　果糖、葡萄糖、淀粉、微晶纤维素。

实验方法

（一）水溶性物料及其混合物的吸湿平衡曲线与临界相对湿度测定

1. 取适量果糖、葡萄糖、果糖－葡萄糖混合物（1∶2，*w/w*），在 40℃干燥箱中干燥 2 小时。

2. 参考附表 1、2，配制相对湿度为 30%、40%、50%、60%、70%、80%、90% 和 100% 的溶液，分别置于一系列干燥容器中，于 25℃恒温箱中平衡 24 小时以上。

3. 将干燥后的样品取适量，分别放入已称重的带盖称量瓶中，轻轻平铺，使样品的厚度约 3mm，盖好瓶盖，称重，打开瓶盖放入已调好湿度的干燥器内。

4. 恒温保存 24 小时，使被测样品中的水分与空气相对湿度达到平衡，取出称量瓶，盖好瓶盖，精密称重，求出增加的重量，计算平衡含水量 %（*w/w*）。

5. 以相对湿度为横坐标，以平衡含水量为纵坐标作图，即可得到样品的吸湿平衡曲线。在吸湿平衡曲线上，吸湿量陡然上升时的相对湿度即为物料的临界相对湿度。

（二）水不溶性物料及其混合物的吸湿平衡曲线测定

1. 取适量淀粉、微晶纤维素、淀粉－微晶纤维素混合物（1∶2，*w/w*），在 40℃干燥箱中干燥 2 小时。

2. 其余操作同上。

（三）注意事项

1. 放入称量瓶的样品不宜过厚，以使物料与空气充分均匀地接触，达到平衡。

2. 不同湿度下，样品的平衡需要一定时间；物料不同，平衡所需的时间不同，有时甚至需要几日。在给定相对湿度下增重（或减重）不变时为平衡状态。本实验恒温保持 24 小时是为了简化实验而设计。

3. 平衡含水量的测定：将样品干燥后作为绝干物料，增重即为平衡吸湿量。平衡水分含量是增重量除以样品吸湿后的总重（绝干物料＋平衡吸湿量）。称重时应尽量快速进行，也可以用水分测定仪直接测平衡水分含量。

实验结果与讨论

1. 结果

（1）将各种物料平衡水分的测定结果记录于表 25-1 和表 25-2 中。

表 25-1　水溶性物料在不同相对湿度下的平衡含水量

相对湿度 /%	30	40	50	60	70	80	90	100
果糖								
葡萄糖								
果糖－葡萄糖								

表 25-2　水不溶性物料在不同相对湿度下的平衡含水量

相对湿度 /%	30	40	50	60	70	80	90	100
淀粉								
微晶纤维素								
淀粉－微晶纤维素								

（2）分别绘出上述 6 种物料的吸湿平衡曲线。

2. 讨论

（1）水溶性物料及其混合物、水不溶性物料及其混合物的吸湿平衡曲线各有什么特征？各自临界相对湿度有何变化？

（2）为什么临界相对湿度是水溶性物料的固有特征？

 思考题

1. 相对湿度和临界相对湿度的区别是什么？

2. 测定吸湿平衡曲线时需要注意什么？

3. 根据物料的吸湿特性，在生产过程中对环境的湿度有何要求？

附表 1　产生各种相对湿度所需硫酸、氢氧化钠、氯化钙在水中浓度（25℃）

相对湿度 /%	H₂SO₄（无水物的重量）/%	NaOH（无水物的重量）/%	CaCl₂（无水物的重量）/%
100	0.0	0.0	0.0
95	11.02	5.54	9.33
90	17.91	9.83	14.95
85	22.88	13.32	19.03
80	26.79	16.10	22.25
75	30.14	18.60	24.95
70	33.09	20.80	27.40
65	35.80	22.80	29.64
60	38.35	24.66	31.73
55	40.75	24.62	33.71
50	43.10	28.16	35.64
45	45.41	29.86	37.61
40	47.71	31.58	39.62
35	50.04	33.38	41.83
30	52.45	35.29	44.36
25	55.01	37.45	/

附表 2　饱和盐溶液在不同温度下产生的相对湿度

盐饱和溶液	25℃ /%	37℃ /%	40℃ /%
K₂Cr₂O₇	98.00		
KNO₃	92.48	91.00	
BaCl₂·2H₂O	90.19		
KCl	84.26		81.70
KBr	80.71	81.00	79.60
NaCl	75.28	75.00	74.70
NaNO₃	73.79		71.50

续表

盐饱和溶液	25℃/%	37℃/%	40℃/%
$NaNO_2$	64.00	62.00	61.50
$NaBr \cdot 2H_2O$	57.00		52.40
$Mg(NO_3)_2 \cdot 6H_2O$	52.86	51.00	
$LiNO_3 \cdot 3H_2O$	47.06		
$K_2CO_3 \cdot 2H_2O$	42.76	41.00	
$MgCl_2 \cdot 6H_2O$	33.00	31.00	
$CH_3COOK \cdot 1.5H_2O$	22.45	23.00	
$LiCl \cdot H_2O$	11.05	11.00	

（李英鹏）

Lab. 25　Determination of Powder Hygroscopicity

Experimental Objectives

1. To master the hygroscopic properties of water-soluble (insoluble) drugs and their mixtures.

2. To be familiar with the drawing method of hygroscopic equilibrium curve and the measurement method of critical relative humidity.

3. To understand the factors that affect the powder hygroscopicity and moisture absorption rate and the improvement measures.

Experimental Principles

Moisture absorption refers to the phenomenon of moisture absorption on a solid surface. When the drug powder is placed in the air with relatively high humidity, different degree of hygroscopicity tends to occur, including the decreasing fluidity, consolidation, wetting, and liquefaction. Hygroscopicity even promotes chemical reactions to reduce the drug's stability.

The hygroscopicity of the powder is related to the air humidity. It is easy to absorb moisture (hygroscopic) in the air with higher humidity, and be dried (air-dried) in dry air until the moisture absorption and drying achieve a dynamic equilibrium. The moisture content in this condition is called balance moisture. The relative humidity (RH) of air is the ratio of the partial pressure of water vapor in the air to the partial pressure of water vapor in saturated air at the same temperature, and it is an important parameter reflecting the air state. The relative humidity of the air is usually from 0 to 100%. The hygroscopic balance curve refers to the ratio of the balance hygroscopic amount and the relative humidity of the powder in the air environment with different relative humidity, which can reflect the hygroscopic characteristics of the powder. The hygroscopic properties of pharmaceutical raw materials and other preparation powders mainly depend on the properties of the powders themselves.

1. Hygroscopicity of Water-soluble Materials　The equilibrium moisture content of water-soluble powder is relatively low in a low relative humidity environment, and it is not hygroscopic. However, when the relative humidity in the air rises to a certain value, the hygroscopicity increases sharply, and the relative humidity at this time is called the critical relative humidity (CRH) of the powder. CRH is an intrinsic characteristic parameter of water-soluble drugs. A smaller CRH indicates that the drug is more hygroscopic. In order to prevent the material from absorbing moisture, the air humidity in the operating environment and storage environment should be below CRH.

According to the Elder hypothesis, the CRH_{AB} of the mixture of water-soluble materials A and B is approximately equal to the product of the two components CRH, regardless of the amount of components, that is, $CRH_{AB} = CRH_A \cdot CRH_B$. It shows that the CRH value of the water-soluble material mixture is lower than that of any of the materials, so it is easier to absorb moisture.

2. Hygroscopicity of Water-insoluble Materials   The hygroscopicity of water-insoluble materials changes slowly when the relative humidity changes, and there is no critical point. Since the equilibrium moisture is adsorbed on the solid surface, it is equivalent to the isothermal adsorption curve of moisture. The hygroscopicity of the water-insoluble material mixture is additive, that is, $CRH_{AB} = CRH_A + CRH_B$.

 Equipments and Materials

1. Equipments   Analytical balances, dryers, thermostats, weighing bottles, etc.

2. Materials   Fructose, glucose, starch, microcrystalline cellulose.

 Experimental Methods

I. Determination of Hygroscopic Equilibrium Curve and Critical Relative Humidity of Water-soluble Materials and Their Mixtures

1. An appropriate amount of fructose, glucose, and a fructose-glucose mixture (1 : 2, w/w) are taken and dried in a drying box at 40℃ for 2 hours.

2. According to Tables 1 and 2, the solutions with relative humidity of 30%, 40%, 50%, 60%, 70%, 80%, 90%, and 100% are prepared and placed in a series of dryers respectively, which are balanced in a 25℃ incubator for more than 24 hours.

3. Take an appropriate amount of the dried samples and put them into a weighing bottle with lid, and spread it gently to make the thickness of the sample about 3mm. Cap the bottle, weigh it, open the bottle and put it in the dryer with adjusted humidity.

4. Keep it at a constant temperature for 24 hours to balance the moisture in the sample and the relative humidity of the air. Take out the weighing bottle, close the cap, and weigh accurately. Calculate the increased weight and calculate the equilibrium moisture content% (w/w).

5. Plot relative humidity as the abscissa and equilibrium moisture content as the ordinate, and obtain the moisture absorption balance curve of the sample. The critical relative humidity of the material refers to the relative humidity when the hygroscopicity increases steeply on the hygroscopic equilibrium curve.

II. Determination of Hygroscopic Equilibrium Curve of Water-insoluble Materials and Their Mixtures

1. An appropriate amount of starch, microcrystalline cellulose, and starch-microcrystalline cellulose mixture (1 : 2, w/w) are taken and dried in a drying cabinet at 40℃ for 2 hours.

2. Other operations are as above.

III. Notes

1. The sample placed in the weighing bottle should not be too thick, so that the material and air are fully and evenly contacted to achieve equilibrium.

2. Under different humidity, it takes time to equilibrate the samples, and the time required for equilibration is different for different materials, sometimes it even take several days. Equilibrium when the weight gain (or weight loss) does not change at a given relative humidity. This experiment is designed at a constant temperature for 24 hours to simplify the experiment.

3. Determination of equilibrium moisture content: After the sample is dried as an absolute dry material, the increase in weight is the equilibrium moisture absorption. The equilibrium moisture content is the added weight divided by the total weight of the sample after moisture absorption (absolutely dry material + equilibrium moisture absorption). Weighing should be performed as quickly as possible. The equilibrium moisture content also can be measured directly with a moisture analyzer.

 Results and Discussions

1. Results

(1) Measurement results of equilibrium moisture of various materials. Records the results in the Table 25–1 and Table 25–2.

Table 25–1   Equilibrium moisture content of water-soluble materials under different relative humidity

Relative humidity/%	30	40	50	60	70	80	90	100
Fructose								
Glucose								
Fructose-glucose								

Table 25–2   Equilibrium moisture content of water-insoluble materials under different relative humidity

Relative humidity/%	30	40	50	60	70	80	90	100
Starch								
Microcrystalline cellulose								
Starch-microcrystalline cellulose								

(2) Draw the hygroscopic equilibrium curve of the above 6 materials respectively.

2. Discussions

(1) What are the characteristics of hygroscopic equilibrium curves of water-soluble materials and their mixtures, and water-insoluble materials and their mixtures? What happens to the respective critical relative humidity?

(2) Why is critical relative humidity an inherent characteristic of water-soluble materials?

 Questions

1. What is the difference between relative humidity and critical relative humidity?

2. What should be paid attention to when determining the hygroscopic equilibrium curve?

3. According to the hygroscopic characteristics of the materials, what are the requirements for the environment humidity in the production process?

Schedule1　Concentrations of sulfuric acid, sodium hydroxide, and calcium chloride in water (25℃) required to produce various relative humidity

Relative humidity/%	H_2SO_4(Anhydrous weight)/%	NaOH(Anhydrous weight)/%	$CaCl_2$(Anhydrous weight)/%
100	0.0	0.0	0.0
95	11.02	5.54	9.33
90	17.91	9.83	14.95
85	22.88	13.32	19.03
80	26.79	16.10	22.25
75	30.14	18.60	24.95
70	33.09	20.80	27.40
65	35.80	22.80	29.64
60	38.35	24.66	31.73
55	40.75	24.62	33.71
50	43.10	28.16	35.64
45	45.41	29.86	37.61
40	47.71	31.58	39.62
35	50.04	33.38	41.83
30	52.45	35.29	44.36
25	55.01	37.45	/

Schedule2　Relative humidity of saturated salt solutions at different temperatures

Saturated salt solutions	25℃/%	37℃/%	40℃/%
$K_2Cr_2O_7$	98.00		
KNO_3	92.48	91.00	
$BaCl_2 \cdot H_2O$	90.19		
KCl	84.26		81.70
KBr	80.71	81.00	79.60
NaCl	75.28	75.00	74.70
$NaNO_3$	73.79		71.50
$NaNO_2$	64.00	62.00	61.50
$NaBr \cdot 2H_2O$	57.00		52.40
$Mg(NO_3)_2 \cdot 6H_2O$	52.86	51.00	
$LiNO_3 \cdot 3H_2O$	47.06		
$K_2CO_3 \cdot 2H_2O$	42.76	41.00	
$MgCl_2 \cdot 6H_2O$	33.00	31.00	
$CH_3COOK \cdot 1.5H_2O$	22.45	23.00	
$LiCl \cdot H_2O$	11.05	11.00	/

实验二十六 流体流变曲线的绘制

 实验目的

1. **掌握** 流体流变曲线的测定原理及绘制方法。
2. **熟悉** 旋转黏度计的使用方法。

实验原理

物质在外力作用下的变形和流动性质，称为流变性。研究流变性的对象往往具有双重性质，它们既具有液体的流动性质，同时也有固体弹性变形的性质。对于液体制剂来说，最重要的流变学特性是黏度。根据流变特性，通常把流体分为两类：一是牛顿流体，遵循牛顿黏性定律；另一类是非牛顿流体，不遵循牛顿黏性定律。

牛顿流体表现为剪切应力与剪切速率成正比，即：$F/A=\eta\,dv/dr$，式中 F/A 为剪切应力，dv/dr 为剪切速率，η 为黏度系数或黏度。牛顿流体的黏度 η 是一个常数，如水、甘油、糖浆都属于牛顿流体。测定牛顿流体黏度常用的仪器有毛细管黏度计（平式和乌式黏度计）和落球黏度计。

非牛顿流体不符合剪切应力和剪切速率成正比的关系，其黏度随剪切应力的变化而变化。如高分子溶液、溶胶、乳浊液、软膏及一些混悬剂等，均属于非牛顿流体。旋转式黏度计可用于牛顿流体或非牛顿流体动力黏度的测定。

把剪切速率（$D=dv/dr$）随剪切应力（$S=F/A$）变化而变化的规律绘制成的曲线称为流变曲线。牛顿流体的流变曲线是通过原点的直线，可以用某一点的黏度绘制流变曲线。非牛顿流体的流变曲线有的不通过原点，且大部分为曲线，流变速率与对应的剪切应力需一一测定后才能绘制出流变曲线。非牛顿流体按流动方式的不同，可分为塑性流体、假塑性流体、胀塑性流体和触变性流体。

流变学对于混悬剂、乳剂、胶体溶液、软膏剂和栓剂等的处方设计、质量评价以及制备工艺的确定都具有重要的指导意义。

实验器材

1. **仪器** 旋转黏度计、杯子、转子、循环水泵、砝码等。
2. **材料** 甘油、羧甲基纤维素钠、蒸馏水等。

实验方法

（一）甘油流变曲线的绘制
本实验使用的旋转黏度计如图 26-1 所示。

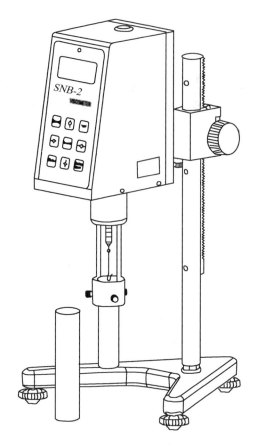

图 26-1 旋转黏度计的结构示意图

Figure 26-1 Structure of a rotary viscometer

1. 将杯子和转子固定位置，通循环水使杯子保持恒温（30℃）。

2. 将甘油倒入杯中标线处，保持循环水温度恒定，使甘油温度不变。

3. 再将砝码挂上后，读出旋转指针的刻度，随后使制动器脱离，记录旋转指针旋转一周的时间，求出旋转的速度（v）。

4. 变换砝码的重量，重复上述操作。

（二）羧甲基纤维素钠水溶液流变曲线的绘制

配制 0.5%、1.0%、3.0% 羧甲基纤维素钠水溶液，如前述固定好杯子和转子，加入羧甲基纤维素水溶液至标线处，保持杯内溶液恒温后，重复上述操作。

实验结果与讨论

1. 对于甘油，依据测定的旋转速度（v）和砝码重量（w）的关系，绘制流变曲线，由直线的斜率求出装置的常数（K_v）。

$$v = K_v \cdot W \cdot 1/\eta \qquad (26\text{-}1)$$

式中，η 为黏度系数；甘油的黏度系数为 624cp（T=30℃）。

2. 各种浓度的羧甲基纤维素钠水溶液的数据，同上述方法处理，当流变曲线为直线时，由上式求出黏度系数。若为非牛顿流体，分析并指出符合哪种类型。

注：非牛顿流体分为塑性流体、假塑性流体和胀塑性流体。塑性流体：曲线不经过原点，在横轴上与剪切应力 S 上的某处有交点，将直线外延至横轴，在 S 上某一点可以得屈服值。假塑性

流体：随着 S 值的增大而黏度下降的流动称为假塑性流动。胀塑性流体：曲线经过原点，且随着剪切应力的增加其黏性也随之增加，表现为向上突起的曲线。

思考题

1. 简述流变学性质对混悬液稳定性的影响。
2. 简述流变学性质对软膏剂处方设计的指导作用。
3. 试说明牛顿流体、塑性流体、假塑性流体、胀塑性流体的区别。

（李英鹏）

Lab. 26 Drawing of Fluid Rheological Curve

 Experimental Objectives

1. To master the measuring principle and drawing method of fluid rheological curve.
2. To be familiar with the use of rotary viscometer.

 Experimental Principles

The deformation and flow properties of matter under external force are called rheology. The research objects of rheology often have dual properties. They have both the fluid flow properties and the solid elastic deformation properties. For liquid formulations, the most important rheological property is viscosity. According to rheological properties, fluids are generally divided into two categories: Newtonian fluid, which follows Newton's law of viscosity; the other is non-Newtonian fluid, which does not follow Newton's law of viscosity.

Newtonian fluid shows that the shear stress is proportional to the shear rate, i.e., $F/A = \eta dv/dz$, where F/A is the shear stress, dv/dz is the shear rate, and η is the viscosity coefficient or viscosity. The viscosity η of a Newtonian fluid is a constant, such as water, glycerin, and syrup belongs to Newtonian fluid. The instruments commonly used to measure the viscosity of Newtonian fluids are capillary viscometers (flat and black viscometers) and falling ball viscometers.

Non-Newtonian fluid do not follow a proportional relationship between shear stress and shear rate, and their viscosity varies with the shear stress. Such as polymer solutions, sols, emulsions, ointments and some suspensions, etc., are non-Newtonian fluid. Rotary viscometer can be used to determine the dynamic viscosity of Newtonian fluid or non-Newtonian fluid.

The curve drawn by the law that the shear rate ($D=dv/dz$) changes with the change of shear stress ($S=F/A$) is called rheological curve. The Newtonian fluid rheological curve is a straight line passing through the origin. The rheological curve can be drawn with the viscosity of a certain point. Some non-Newtonian fluid rheological curves do not pass through the origin, and most of them are curves. The rheological curve can only be drawn after the rheological rate and the corresponding shear stress are measured one by one. Non-Newtonian fluids can be divided into plastic fluids, pseudoplastic fluids, dilatant fluids, and thixotropic fluids according to their flow patterns.

Rheology plays important roles in prescription design, quality evaluation and preparation process of suspensions, emulsions, colloidal solutions, ointments and suppositories.

 Equipments and Materials

1. Equipments Rotary viscometer, cup, rotor, circulating water pump, weight, etc.

2. Materials Glycerin, sodium carboxymethyl cellulose, distilled water, etc.

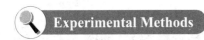 **Experimental Methods**

I. Drawing of Glycerin Rheological Curve

The experimental rotary viscometer is shown in the Figure 26–1.

(1) Fix the cup and the rotor in a fixed position and keep the cup at a constant temperature (30℃) by circulating water.

(2) Pour glycerin into the marked line in the cup, and keep the glycerin temperature constant by keeping the circulating water temperature constant.

(3) After hanging the weight, read out the scale of the rotary pointer, and then release the brake, record the time of one rotation of the rotary pointer, and find out the speed of rotation (v).

(4) Change the weight of the weights and repeat the above operation.

II. Drawing of Rheological Curve of Sodium Carboxymethyl Cellulose Aqueous Solution

Prepare 0.5%, 1.0%, 3.0% sodium carboxymethyl cellulose aqueous solution, fix the cup and rotor as described above, add the sodium carboxymethyl cellulose aqueous solution to the marked line, and keep the solution in the cup constant temperature, then repeat the above operation.

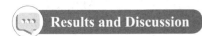 **Results and Discussion**

1. Results For glycerin, draw a rheological curve based on the relationship between the measured rotational speed (v) and the weight of the weight (w), and determine the constant (K_v) of the device from the slope of the straight line.

$$v=K_v \cdot W \cdot 1/\eta \tag{26-1}$$

Where, η is the viscosity coefficient; the viscosity coefficient of glycerin is 624cp (T=30℃).

2. Discussions The data of various concentrations of sodium carboxymethyl cellulose aqueous solution are processed with the above method. When the rheological curve is a straight line, the viscosity coefficient is obtained from the above formula. For non-Newtonian fluids, analyze the appropriate fluid type.

Notes: Non-Newtonian fluids are divided into plastic fluids, pseudoplastic fluids, and dilatant fluids. Plastic fluid: The curve does not pass through the origin, but interacts somewhere on the S-axis of shear stress on the horizontal axis. The straight line is extended to the horizontal axis, and the yield value can be obtained at some point on the S-axis. Pseudoplastic fluid: The flow whose viscosity decreases as the S value increases is called pseudoplastic flow. Dilatant fluid: The curve passes through the origin and its viscosity increases with increasing shear stress, manifesting as a curve protruding upward.

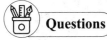 **Questions**

1. Briefly describe the influence of rheological properties on the stability of suspensions.

2. Briefly describe the guiding role of rheological properties in the design of ointment prescription.

3. Explain the difference between Newtonian fluid, plastic fluid, pseudoplastic fluid, and dilatant fluid.

实验二十七　软膏锥入度的测定

实验目的

1. **掌握**　软膏锥入度的测定原理及方法。
2. **熟悉**　锥入度仪的结构及使用方法。

实验原理

锥入度系指利用自由落体运动，在25℃下，将一定质量的锥体由锥入度仪释放，测定锥体释放后5秒内刺入供试品的深度，用于控制软膏剂、眼膏剂及其基质材料等半固体物质的软硬度和黏稠度，以使其可挤出性、涂布延展性符合使用要求，提高患者用药的依从性。一般稠度大的样品锥入度小，产品从软管中挤出时阻力大，在皮肤上的涂布延展性不佳，不便于使用；稠度小的样品锥入度大，易于挤出、涂布和延展，但稠度太小则易于流动，产品挤出、涂敷时不易控制，难于黏附固定于给药位置。因此，锥入度对于软膏剂的处方设计、质量评价以及制备工艺的确定都具有重要的指导意义。

实验器材

1. **仪器**　锥入度计、锥体、样品杯等。
2. **材料**　水杨酸油脂性软膏、水杨酸乳膏、水杨酸水溶性软膏。

实验方法

（一）锥入度计结构

1. 仪器工作台结构　实验用锥入度计由水平底座、支柱、水平升降台、释放装置、水平调节仪、显示装置等组成，如图27-1所示。水平调节仪用于保证锥杆垂直度，使锥尖与样品杯中心保持一致；水平升降台能准确调节锥尖，使锥尖与待测样品表面恰好接触；释放装置能自动释放锥体，即时测出锥体5秒所刺入深度，并在锥入度值显示装置上显示结果。

2. 锥体结构　锥体由圆锥体和锥尖组成，表面光滑，共有三种可供选择：Ⅰ号锥体质量为102.5g±0.05g，配套锥杆质量为47.5g±0.05g；Ⅱ号锥体质量为22.5g±0.025g，配套锥杆质量为15g±0.025g；Ⅲ号锥体及锥杆总质量为9.38g±0.025g。三种锥体形状尺寸如图27-2所示。

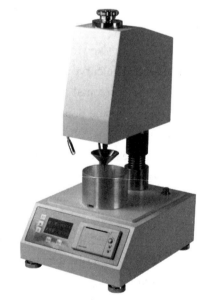

图 27-1　锥入度计
Figure 27-1　Cone penetration meter

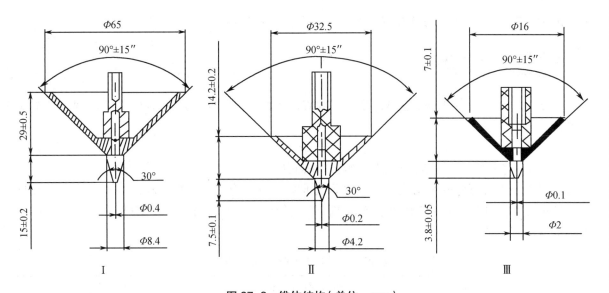

图 27-2　锥体结构（单位：mm）

Figure 27-2　Cone structure（unit：mm）

3. 样品杯　为平底圆筒，不同型号锥体配套使用不同型号样品杯，Ⅰ～Ⅲ号锥体配套使用样品杯的形状尺寸如图 27-3 所示。根据样品量选择适当锥体进行测定，推荐选用Ⅱ号锥体和样品杯进行本项目测定。

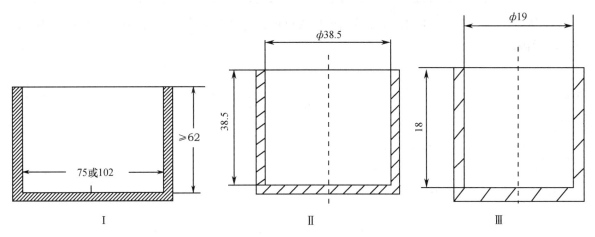

图 27-3　样品杯（单位：mm）

Figure 27-3　Specimens cups（unit：mm）

（二）样品锥入度的测定

1. 测定前，调试仪器装置，使锥尖恰好落于中心位置。

2. 供试品按下述方法之一处理。

（1）将供试品小心装满样品杯，并高出样品杯上沿约 2mm，避免产生气泡，在平坦的台面上振动样品杯约 5 分钟，除去可能混入的气泡。

（2）按照标准规定将供试品熔融后，小心装满样品杯，并高出样品杯上沿约 2mm，避免产生气泡。装好样品后，在 25℃ ±0.5℃放置 24 小时。

3. 刮平表面，将样品杯置锥入度计的底座上，调节位置使锥体尖端与供试品的表面刚好接触，并控制杯子保持恒温（25℃ ±0.5℃）。

4. 迅速释放Ⅱ号锥体（应在 0.1 秒内完成下落动作）并维持 5 秒后，读出锥入深度（r），以锥入度单位表示，1 个锥入度单位等于 0.1mm。重复测定 3 次。

实验结果与讨论

1. 结果 记录 4 种水杨酸软膏的锥入深度值，依据公式（27-1）将测定值换算成使用 I 号锥体的推测值。

$$p=2r+5 \qquad\qquad (27-1)$$

式中，p 为 I 号锥体的推测值；r 为 II 号锥体的实测值。

结果以 3 次推测值的平均值表示。如单次推测值与平均值的相对偏差大于 3.0%，应重复试验，结果以 6 次推测值的平均值表示（表 27-1），并计算相对标准偏差（RSD）。6 次推测值的相对标准偏差应小于 5.0%。

表 27-1 软膏锥入度的测定结果

水杨酸软膏样品	锥入深度值 /mm						p/mm	RSD/%
	1	2	3	4	5	6		
油脂性基质								
O/W 型乳膏								
W/O 型乳膏								
水溶性基质								

2. 讨论 对比不同基质制备所得软膏的锥入度值，讨论各基质对软膏黏稠性及涂布性等的影响及其原因。

思考题

1. 试述锥入度与软膏性能的相关性。
2. 软膏锥入度大小受哪些因素影响？
3. 锥入度如何指导软膏剂的处方设计？

（谢兴亮）

Lab.27 Determination of Cone Penetration of Ointment

 Experimental Objectives

1. To master testing principles and methods for cone penetration of ointment.
2. To be familiar with the structure and usage of cone penetration meter.

 Experimental Principles

Cone penetration refers to determine the depth of penetration into the sample within 5 seconds after releasing a certain mass of cone from the penetrometer by free-fall motion at 25℃, which is used for controlling softness and viscosity of semi-solid substances such as ointments, eye ointments and their base materials, so as to make their extrudability and coating ductility meet the use requirements and improve patients' medication compliance. Generally, the cone penetration of the sample with higher viscosity is smaller, and the resistance is larger when it is extruded from the hose and coating ductility is not good, so it is not easy to use; while the sample with a smaller viscosity has a larger cone penetration, it is easy to be extruded and extended. However, the sample with too small viscosity flows easily, and is difficult to control its extrusion and coating, and it is also difficult to adhere and fix in the dosing location. Therefore, the cone penetration has important guiding significance for the formulation design, quality evaluation and preparation process of ointment.

 Equipments and Materials

1. Equipments　Cone penetration meter, cone, sample cups, etc.

2. Materials　Salicylic acid greasy ointment, salicylic acid cream, salicylic acid water-soluble ointment.

 Experimental Methods

I. Structure of Cone Penetration Meter

1. Structure of workbench　The cone penetration meter is composed of a horizontal base, pillar, horizontal lifting platform, release device, horizontal adjusting instrument, display device, etc (Figure 27–1). Horizontal adjuster is used to ensure the verticality of cone rod, so that the cone tip is consistent with the center of sample cups. Horizontal elevator is used to adjust the cone accurately so that its tip is in contact with the surface of the specimen. Release device can automatically release the cone and instantly measure the penetration depth of cone in 5 seconds, and display the result of cone penetration value on the display device.

2. Structure of cone　Cone is composed of cone body and tip with a smooth surface. There are three types: The mass of No. I cone is 102.5g ± 0.05g, and the mass of its matching rod is 47.5g ± 0.05g; the mass of No. II cone is 22.5g ± 0.025g, and the mass of its matching rod is 15g ± 0.025g; the total mass of No. III cone and rod is 9.38g ± 0.025g. The shapes and sizes of three cones are shown in the Figure 27–2.

3. Sample cup　It is a flat-bottomed cylinder. There are three models of sample cups respectively matching three types of cones. The shapes and sizes of the sample cups are as shown in the Figure 27–3. According to the sample volume, select an appropriate cone for determination. It is recommended to use cone II and cup II for the determination of this experiment.

II. Determination of Cone Penetration of Samples

1. Debug the instrument before the measurement so that the cone tip is exactly at the central location.

2. The testing sample is treated as one of the following methods.

(1) Carefully fill the sample cup with the testing sample and raise it approximately 2mm above the upper edge of the cup to avoid air bubbles and shake the cup on a flat table for 5 minutes to remove possible bubbles.

(2) After the testing sample has been melted as specified in the standard, fill the sample cup carefully and raise it approximately 2mm above the upper edge of the cup to avoid bubbles. After the samples are loaded, place them at 25℃ ± 0.5℃ for 24h.

3. Slick the surface, place the sample cup on the base of cone penetration meter, adjust the position so that the cone tip just contacts with the surface of a test sample, and control the temperature of the cup to be kept constant (25℃ ±0.5℃).

4. Read the penetration depth (*r*) of cone after quickly releasing cone II and maintaining it for 5 seconds (Drop action should be completed within 0.1 second). It is expressed in cone units, 1 cone unit is equal to 0.1mm. Repeat the determination 3 times.

??? Results and Discussions

1. Results　Record the values of cone penetration depth of four salicylic acid ointments and convert the measured values to the presumed values using cone I according to the following formula.

$$p=2r+5 \qquad\qquad (27\text{--}1)$$

Where, *p* is the presumed value of cone I and *r* is the measured value of cone II .

The result is presented as the mean of three presumed values. If the relative deviation from the mean is greater than 3.0%, the test should be repeated and the result is expressed as the mean of the six predicted values (Table 27–1), and the relative standard deviation (*RSD*) should be calculated and be less than 5.0%.

Table 27–1　Determination results of cone penetration of ointment

Salicylic acid ointment samples	Value of cone penetration depth/mm						*p*/mm	*RSD*/%
	1	2	3	4	5	6		
Greasy base								
O/W cream								
W/O cream								
Water soluble base								

2. Discussion Compare the cone penetration values of ointments prepared from different bases and discuss the effects of each base on the viscosity and coatability of ointments and its reasons.

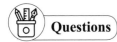 **Questions**

1. Describe the correlation between cone penetration and ointment performance.
2. What factors affect the values of cone penetration of ointments?
3. How does cone penetration guide the formulation design of ointments?

参考文献

［1］崔福德.药剂学［M］.7版.北京：人民卫生出版社，2012.

［2］方亮.药剂学［M］.8版.北京：人民卫生出版社，2016.

［3］崔福德.药剂学实验指导［M］.3版.北京：人民卫生出版社，2011.

［4］李超英，李范珠.药剂学实验［M］.北京：中国中医药出版社，2013.

［5］张兆旺.中药药剂学［M］.2版.北京：中国中医药出版社，2007.

［6］周建平.药剂学实验与指导［M］.北京：化学工业出版社，2012.

［7］Loyd V. Allen Jr., Nicholas G. Popovich, Howard C. Ansel, etc. 安塞尔药物剂型给药系统［M］.
9版.王浩，侯惠民，等，译.北京：科学出版社，2012.